HUMAN
SEXUALITY

HUMAN
SEXUALITY

a health practitioner's text

edited by
RICHARD GREEN, M.D.

Professor, Department of Psychiatry
and Behavioral Science
Professor, Department of Psychology
State University of New York at Stony Brook
Stony Brook, New York

with 19 contributors

The Williams & Wilkins Company
BALTIMORE

Made in the United States of America

Reprinted 1976

Library of Congress Cataloging in Publication Data

Green, Richard, 1936-
    Human sexuality: a health practitioner's text.

    1. Sexual disorders. 2. Sex (Biology). 3. Sex (Psychology). I. Title. [DNLM: 1. Sex behavior—Sex manuals. HQ21 G797h]
RC556.G73 1975   616.6   74-10562
ISBN 0-683-03551-7

Reprinted 1978

Copyright Acknowledgments

Chapter 9. The material of this chapter, slightly adapted, first appeared in a Symposium on Sex Assignment and Reassignment: Intersex and Gender Identity Disorders (Jon K. Meyer, guest editor), *Clinics in Plastic Surgery,* 1:215-222 and 271-274. W. B. Saunders Company, Philadelphia, 1974. Used with permission of W. B. Saunders Company.

Chapter 15. "Treating Sexual Dysfunction: The Solo Male Clinician," by C. E. Vincent has been adapted, by the Author and Editor from *Sexual and Marital Health: The Physician as a Consultant,* by C. E. Vincent. Copyright 1973, McGraw-Hill. Used with permission of McGraw-Hill Book Company.

Grant Acknowledgments

Chapter 1. This research is partially based on work supported by a Grant from the Commonwealth Fund.

Chapter 3. This work was supported in part by funds from the Ford Foundation and in part by funds from Public Health Service Grants HD-05179 and HD-05853 of the National Institute of Child Health and Human Development.

Chapter 5. This chapter derives, in part, from a study supported by NIMH Grant MH 15527.

Chapter 7. This research was supported by NIMH Grants MH 31-739, MH 24-305, and the Foundations' Fund for Research in Psychiatry Grant G69-471.

Chapter 9. This study was supported by the Grant Foundation, New York, and United States Public Health Service Grant HD 00325.

Chapter 12. This work was supported in part by Social and Rehabilitation Service Research and Training Grant 16-P-56810.

Composed and printed at the
Waverly Press, Inc.
Mt. Royal and Guilford Aves.
Baltimore, Md. 21202, U.S.A.

Preface

THE MAKING OF ANOTHER TEXT

I swore I wouldn't edit another book. I had co-edited *Transsexualism and Sex Reassignment* in 1969, and it was a nightmare. My previous idea of an editor's task was to neatly pile up a set of manuscripts written by others, fire a staple gun into the left margin at appropriate intervals, and signal the task as completed.

First, I learned that to obtain commitments from people to write a textbook chapter is not easy—by the time an investigator arrives at the career point in which "expert" status is achieved, that person is so overcommitted to writing, lecturing, and further research, that the invitation is received as a chore, not flattery.

Second, two writers rarely write in the same style, and when collating chapters by a multitude of authors, someone has to align their styles so the book comes together into a cohesive pattern. Guess who's task *that* is?

Third, while everyone promises to have chapters in on a certain date, the Editor grows increasingly nervous as not only don't manuscripts *pour* in, but they barely *dribble*. The frantic Editor then attempts to reestablish contact with the erstwhile contributors. One-third are on an overseas sabbatical; one-third are three chapters behind on commitments made prior to this; and one-third totally forgot about the book. After 3 years of assembling *Transsexualism and Sex Reassignment,* I swore I would *never* edit another book.

I did not, however, promise not to *write* one. This, it appeared to me, couldn't be any worse than editing one, since the Editor in the final analysis re-writes much of the material anyway and receives little credit for the toil. So with naive enthusiasm I agreed to write my own.

One day in 1973, my office floor was covered with hundreds of page proofs of *Sexual Identity Conflict in Children and Adults.* I had been working at this relatively simple task only 4 years now. I had re-written page after page, and had seen the scrawled, then typewritten pages go to copy-editing, only to be re-written again. At last, one day they had made it to galley form. They were type set. Done! My euphoria had been premature. I had forgotten about *one more* reading of every page, every word, every *letter.* The *page* proofs. Never again would I write a book.

While I was casting about in this tidal wave of page proofs the phone rang. It was the Chairman of my Department, "Jolly" West. Flabbergasted at his calling (this phenomenon averaged once a year), I scurried to his office. There I was introduced to Steve Thaler, representing James Gallagher of Williams and Wilkins. Jolly said the publishers were interested in finding someone to edit a book which would serve as a text for medical school human sexuality courses. Since I had chaired the course that year, Jolly suggested Thaler and I talk. Hardly the best of timing.

I gave Thaler 10 minutes and went back to my page proofs. Two days later the page proofs were on their way back to the publisher (for some reason, publishers, though they take 6 months to get proofs to an author, give authors only 48 hours to return them, lest every incredible printer's mistake be indelibly inked for posterity).

The thought of a textbook on human sexuality for medical students and doctors began to preoccupy and then to excite me. There really wasn't any such text. I began to think of topic areas in our course and others—such as sexuality in the paraplegic, sexuality in the mentally retarded, the treatment of sexual incompatibilities in couples, how female patients feel about having a pelvic, what it's like to be a homosexual physician, etc. There really wasn't anything available under one cover, let alone in scattered sources. I realized that I was friendly with people whose work in these areas I knew and relied on, and that their special knowledge hadn't been put together into a practical text. Ninety-five medical schools teaching human sexuality and no appropriate book! Remarkable! At a time when we are drowning in publication redundancy, a publishing vacuum.

Then, the memory of the first editing ordeal returned to haunt me. But, by then (1973), I had become experienced in another type of editing. For 2 years I had been Editor of a journal: *The Archives of Sexual Behavior.* In a self-deluding moment, though the old staple gun fantasy of book editing was long extinguished, I considered editing a book no worse than bringing out the next journal issue.

So deluded, I proceeded. However, with this book, I invoked a different editing strategy. I contacted the people I considered the experts in their subfield of human sexuality. I presented the challenge—believe it or not—a genuine textbook void, an opportunity to make a significant input to medical education. Everyone was offered a cut of the pie: we would all share in royalties. If the book sold 100 copies, we'd each buy a glass of wine and drink it simultaneously, in separate cities. If it sold 10,000 copies, we'd all fly somewhere and drink it together.

A manuscript deadline was presented. It was a realistic gestation period—9 months. During the last trimester, reminder letters began to besiege contributors at an accelerating rate. Guilt levels rose. Manuscripts began to arrive.

A list of all contributors who had agreed to participate was sent to each contributor. Final deadlines were given and, if not met, the book would go to press without that person's chapter. Embarrassment levels rose. The remaining manuscripts arrived.

Two contributors opted for an alternative. What was wanted had recently been approximated in another paper. I agreed to revise these works to accommodate the text's style and purpose. The other 16 chapters were written specifically for this text.

Each manuscript was edited and the reworked version returned to the authors. They are still my friends. And I am grateful as hell to them. But I swear, I'll *never* . . .

Richard Green

Contributors

ALAN P. BELL, Ph.D.
Senior Research Psychologist, Institute for Sex Research, Indiana University, Bloomington, Indiana

MAE BIGGS, M.S.
Reproductive Biology Research Foundation, St. Louis, Missouri

JULIUS C. BUTLER, Jr., M.D.
Assistant Professor of Obstetrics and Gynecology, University of Minnesota, Minneapolis, Minnesota

THEODORE M. COLE, M.D.
Associate Professor, Department of Physical Medicine and Rehabilitation, University of Minnesota, Minneapolis, Minnesota

MILTON DIAMOND, Ph.D.
Professor, Anatomy, and Reproductive Biology, School of Medicine, University of Hawaii, Honolulu, Hawaii

R. KURT EBERT, Ph.D.
Associate in Psychiatry, Research Director, Center for the Study of Sex Education in Medicine, University of Pennsylvania School of Medicine, Philadelphia, Pennsylvania

RICHARD GREEN, M.D.
Professor, Department of Psychiatry and Behavioral Science, Professor, Department of Psychology, State University of New York at Stony Brook, Stony Brook, New York

JUDY E. HALL, Ph.D.
Assistant Professor of Experimental Psychology and Staff Psychologist, Center for Developmental and Learning Disorders, University of Alabama Medical Center, Birmingham, Alabama

HAROLD I. LIEF, M.D.
Professor of Psychiatry, Director, Center for the Study of Sex Education in Medicine, University of Pennsylvania School of Medicine, Philadelphia, Pennsylvania

REVEREND TED McILVENNA, M.Div.
National Sex Forum, Genesis Church and Ecumenical Center, San Francisco, California

HENRY D. MESSER, M.D., F.A.C.S.
Chief, Neurosurgery, Harlem Hospital Medical Center of Columbia University, Private Practice of Neurosurgery, New York, New York

JOHN MONEY, Ph.D.
Professor of Medical Psychology, Associate Professor of Pediatrics, The Johns Hopkins University School of Medicine, Baltimore, Maryland

RONALD PION, M.D.
Professor, Obstetrics and Gynecology, School of Medicine, and Population Studies and Family Planning, School of Public Health, University of Hawaii, Honolulu, Hawaii

IRA L. REISS, Ph.D.
Professor, Department of Sociology, Director, Family Study Center, University of Minnesota, Minneapolis, Minnesota

DIANE S. FORDNEY SETTLAGE, M.D., M.S.
Assistant Professor of Obstetrics and Gynecology, Head, Pediatric and Adolescent Gynecology Clinic, Head, Sexual Function Clinic, University of Southern California School of Medicine, Los Angeles, California

RICHARD SPITZ, M.D.
Reproductive Biology Research Foundation, St. Louis, Missouri

HERBERT E. VANDERVOORT, M.D.
Faculty Member in Charge, Human Sexuality Program, School of Medicine, University of California, San Francisco, California

CLARK E. VINCENT, Ph.D.
Director, Behavioral Sciences Center, Bowman Gray School of Medicine, Winston-Salem, North Carolina

NATHANIEL N. WAGNER, Ph.D.
Professor of Psychology, and Obstetrics and Gynecology, University of Washington, Seattle, Washington

Contents

chapter

1

Is sex education necessary for medical students, physicians, and other health science professionals? Is a separate course needed? Another text?

Do not medical people by virtue of their general educational level and their special training in biology have sufficient knowledge to answer patient questions about sex? Do not the standard texts and courses cover sexual anatomy and physiology, sex history taking, sex behavior and heart attacks, sex during late pregnancy, sex after spinal cord injury, how to assign sex to intersexed infants, the sex life of the mentally retarded, attitudinal issues about contraception and abortion, how to do a pelvic examination in a female, treatment of sexual failure in men and women, what constitutes the range of sexual behavior in typical individuals, and the life style of homo-sexual patients and physicians? As observed in the preface, it is the absence of coverage of these areas in readily accessible form which has created the demand for this volume.

The second half of the 20th century has experienced a public explosion of interest in sexuality. Sex-theme books have dominated the best-seller lists of recent years: Everything You Always Wanted to Know About Sex, The Sensuous Woman, The Sensuous Man, Human Sexual Response, Human Sexual Inadequacy , *and* The Joy of Sex. *Films with major sexual themes have been produced and widely attended:* Carnal Knowledge, Last Tango In Paris, *and* Deep Throat, *Sexuality is openly discussed; it is within the public domain. With this change has come the demand for accurate information and personal sexual fulfillment.*

Dilemmas have also evolved. New methods for separating intercourse from pregnancy and pregnancy from childbirth, the growing concept of a wide

Why Sex Education
for Medical Students?

R. KURT EBERT, Ph.D.

HAROLD I. LIEF, M.D.

variety of sexual practices as healthy forms of self-expression, generational differences in value systems between parents and teenagers, and the political activities of the Gay Liberation and Women's Movements have convulsed contemporary culture.

Physicians remain the professionals from whom factual information and help are most often expected. Have currently practicing physicians been prepared to fill that role? Hardly. Chapter 1 briefly documents the need for the incorporation of sex education as a formal component of medical education. Material follows to meet better the public need.

Editor

During the past decade traditional attitudes toward marriage and sexuality have undergone serious challenge. With sex no longer a taboo topic, every conceivable difficulty concerning sexuality is being brought by patients to the physician's office—questions concerning sex education, masturbation, homosexuality, sexual functioning, and, most frequently, problems of sexual inadequacy and sexual incompatibility.

While Masters and Johnson (1970) believe that a minimum of 50% of all married couples are troubled by sexual problems, Burnap and Golden (1967) have shown that the number of sexual problems encountered in a physician's practice is directly related to the physician's comfort with the topic. Thus over 66% of physicians who routinely obtain a sexual history from their patients identify significant sexual problems in at least 50% of the patients who consult them. On the other hand, over 75% of those physicians who do not actively inquire about their patients' sex lives estimate that less than 10% of their patients have sexual problems.

Because the topic of sexuality involves strong feelings and deeply rooted value orientations, both the teaching and learning of human sexuality are more complex than are most other areas of medical education. The mastery of a body of factual information is simply inadequate to effectively deal with the variety of sexual problems with which physicians are constantly confronted. Knowledge of gross anatomy does not confer on the physician knowledge of how to help a teenager to manage strong sexual feelings and desires; knowledge of the physiology of conception and procreation does not include methods of handling the problems of young married couples who are sexually frustrated; knowing how to deliver a baby does not mean that a doctor can rescue a middle-aged man who is panicky because of failing sexual powers.

The need to be able to deal effectively with the sex problems of patients is recognized by physicians after a relatively short time in practice. Sex problems constitute a significant part of the emotional problems of living: in family life a primary motivating force is a warm, secure marital relationship, and sex makes a unique contribution to the maintenance of this relationship.

Briefly summarized, the tasks of the effective physician-counselor in dealing with sexual problems are: 1) Be comfortable with sexual topics and put the patient at ease. 2) Listen well and know how to take a sexual history. 3) Always show concern for the patient's feelings; do nothing to increase the patient's shame and embarrassment. 4) Judge whether the sexual problems uncovered in the history taking are within the competence of the physician-counselor. 5) If they are within the physician-counselor's competence, set up a plan of treatment with the patient's full knowledge and consent. 6) If they are not within the physician-counselor's competence, refer the patient to another professional person who has the required knowledge and skills (Lief, 1974).

The key dimension in becoming a comfortable and effective physician-sex counselor is an increased awareness of one's own feelings and attitudes about sexuality: if one has a clear concept of just what it is that he or she believes in, one is less apt to unwittingly impose those values on the patient or have them affect clinical judgment and management. The physician who is unable to accept premarital intercourse under any circumstances is a poor choice for the single girl who is looking for contraceptive help. The physician who condemns extramarital sex, irrespective of the circumstances, may "preach" to his "sinful" patient and, in this fashion, sabotage rapport. Similarly, a physician may suggest masturbation to a patient not ready to accept such counsel.

In a recent survey conducted by the Center for the Study of Sex Education in Medicine at the University of Pennsylvania School of Medicine, 68% of medical sex educators reported that attitude modification was the primary need of their students; 18% reported that the acquisition of knowledge was the most important need; and nearly 15% reported that the development of treatment skills was most important (Lief and Ebert, 1974).

Data from the nationwide study of medical students' sexual knowledge and attitudes, currently in process in our Center, graphically illustrate why medical educators rank student needs the way they do. Using the Sex Knowledge and Attitude Test (SKAT) as our main data-gathering instrument, we have found that although medical students' attitudes in the areas of premarital and extramarital heterosexual relations differ little from those of non-medical undergraduate students, medical students are more rejecting of sexual myths and more knowledgeable. However, in comparison to non-medical graduate students, medical students are significantly more conservative on all sexual attitudes measured and significantly *less* knowledgeable.

Table 1 presents the average SKAT attitude and knowledge scores we have obtained from a sample of over 4,800 college, graduate, and medical students tested during 1971 and 1972. The SKAT contains four attitudinal scales in addition to the knowledge score:

HR (Heterosexual Relations Scale) measures an individual's attitudes toward premarital and extramarital heterosexual encounters. Individuals with high HR scores (above 60) regard premarital and extramarital sexual relations as acceptable or even desirable, and as potentially benefiting rather than harming the marital relationship. Scores below 40 on the HR scale imply conservative attitudes regarding the acceptability of premarital and extra-marital sexual relations.

TABLE 1:
SKAT scores for medical students and non-medical
college and graduate students

| | Attitude Scales | | | | Knowledge | |
	HR	SM	A	M	Score	N
Medical students	49.29	49.63	48.38	49.60	50.25	3,474
College students	48.77	45.86	46.84	47.55	41.03	990
Graduate students	51.90	54.54	50.91	52.30	53.90	358

Both the attitude and the knowledge scores presented in Table 1 are specially derived "deviation" scores, which relate an individual's or group's performance on the SKAT to the average performance of a specially gathered normative sample of first- to fourth-year medical students. Through statistical conversion the "average performance" of this normative sample was equated with a score of 50. Under this conversion system 68% of all medical students received scores ranging from 40 to 60; over 96% received scores between 30 and 70. Scores outside of these ranges were rare.

SM (Sexual Myths Scale) measures an individual's acceptance or rejection of commonly held sexual misconceptions, taboos, and fallacies. High scores (above 60) indicate a rejection of these misconceptions. The lower the score, the greater the degree of acceptance of popular misconceptions.

The A (Abortion) Scale measures an individual's general social, medical, and legal feelings toward abortion. High scores (above 60) imply an orientation which sees abortion as an acceptable form of birth control, to be permitted whenever desired by the pregnant woman; the lower the score (below 40), the greater the negative feeling about abortion.

The M (Masturbatory) attitude scale measures an individual's attitudes toward masturbation. Individuals with high scores (above 60) view autoerotic stimulation as healthy and acceptable. Low scores (below 40) imply an orientation which views masturbation as an unacceptable and unhealthy practice. The lower the score, the greater the negative feeling about masturbation.

TABLE 2:
Approximate percentile ranks of medical students and
non-medical college and graduate students for the
SKAT attitude and knowledge scores

| | Attitude Scales | | | | Knowledge |
	HR	SM	A	M	Score
Medical students	50	50	50	50	50
College students	45	34	38	40	19
Graduate students	57	67	54	59	69

Table 2 presents a comparison of the average SKAT scores from Table 1 in terms of percentile rank.

A selection of some of the SKAT items will highlight the need for medical sex education. Thirty five percent of female medical students and 37% of male medical students do not believe that "impotence is almost always a psychogenic disorder." Thirty five percent of male medical students and 51% of female medical students believe that "one of the immediate results of castration in the adult male is impotence." Twenty five percent of male medical students and 35% of female medical students believe that "only a small minority of all married couples ever experience mouth-genital sex-play." Thirty one percent of female medical students and 36% of male medical students do not believe that "25% of men over the age of 70 have an active sexual life." Fifteen percent of female medical students and 15% of male medical students still believe that "certain conditions of mental and emotional instability are demonstrably caused by masturbation." The latter is a significant improvement over Greenbank's finding (1961) reported more than a decade ago that 50% of medical students thought that masturbation is causally related to mental illness. Yet our finding that 15% of medical students still believe this ancient myth is a cause for continued concern.

Many obstacles, primarily attitudinal, have retarded the universal inclusion of sex education in medical school curricula. Nevertheless, the pressures of social change and new sexual life styles have brought about an almost unrecognized revolution in medical education. In 1960 only three medical schools offered formal courses in sex education. By 1973 almost all medical schools in the United States were involved in the teaching of human sexuality in the medical school curricula.

Why a sex education course for medical students? Because physicians are regarded by the lay public as experts on sex. More people seek help for emotional and psychological problems from non-psychiatric physicians than they do from any other single source of professional help other than the clergy.

But are physicians experts on sex? The weight of current evidence indicates they are not. Sexual behavior is intimately involved with the psychological and emotional aspects of life, an area in which physicians are woefully ignorant. Physicians and medical students are relatively ignorant about sexual behavior from even a purely descriptive or phenomenological point of view. In short, many physicians are not much better informed than the patients they counsel. Only when it comes to the anatomy and the physiology of the sex apparatus can physicians, at least relatively speaking, claim to be experts.

Obviously, this is not enough. Other than the care of the dying patient, there is no other place in medical practice where attitudes play such an important role in the management of clinical problems. Since everyone has a set of beliefs and preferences based on personal experience and judgments, it is unrealistic to expect a physician to be free of individual biases. What we must try to do is not free the physician from those beliefs, but rather to develop an awareness of his or her own set of values. It is only when the medical student or physician has a clear concept of what he or she believes in that the clinician will be able to keep private values from unwittingly affecting medical judgment and management.

REFERENCES

Athanasiou, R. 1973. A Review of Public Attitudes on Sexual Issues. In *Contemporary Sexual Behavior: Critical Issues in the 1970's* (J. Zubin and J. Money, eds.). Baltimore: The Johns Hopkins University Press.

Burnap, D.W., and Golden, J.S. 1967. Sexual Problems in Medical Practice. Med. Educ. 42:1967. 673-680.

Greenbank, R. K. 1961. Are Medical Students Learning Psychiatry? Pa. Med. J. 64: 989-992.

Lief, H. I. 1974. Sexual Knowledge, Attitudes, and Behavior of Medical Students: Implications for Medical Practice. In *Marital and Sexual Counseling in Medical Practice* (D. W. Abse and L. M. R. Louden, eds.). New York: Harper and Row.

Lief, H. I. and Ebert, R. K. A Survey of Sex Education in United States Medical Schools. Paper presented at the World Health Organization Symposium on "Education and Treatment in Human Sexuality: The Training of Health Professionals." February 4 to 12, 1974, Geneva, Switzerland.

Masters, W. H. and Johnson, V. E. 1970. *Human Sexual Inadequacy*. Boston: Little, Brown and Co.

Pauly, I. B. 1971. Human Sexuality in Medical Education and Practice. Aust., N.Z. Psychiatry. 5: 206-219.

Reiss, I. 1967. *The Social Context of Premarital Sexual Permissiveness*. New York: Holt, Rinehart and Winston.

chapter

2

Should a sex history be part of the general medical history? Unless the patient's chief complaint is in the area of sexuality, is specific questioning appropriate? Should this intimate part of a patient's life be better left to psychiatrists and psychologists?

If a sex history is to be taken, is the technique any different from questioning about other aspects of health? Are there ways in which questions can be asked which reduce patient defensiveness? Are there target areas for questioning which resonate with problems of the average patient? The next chapter addresses itself to these questions.

Editor

Taking a Sexual History

RICHARD GREEN, M.D.

Sex History Taking: Why?

Emotional health and physical health are so interwoven that to neglect the emotional is inadequate coverage of the physical. Sexual health is so integral to both that to ignore the sexual is poor patient care. Thus, medical history taking is incomplete without a comprehensive sex history. Conflicts over sexuality can result in depression, anxiety, and alcholism. Depression, anxiety, and alcohol abuse lead to reduced sex drive and inadequate sexual functioning. Diabetes can lead to male impotence; postoperative surgical adhesions can result in painful female intercourse; Klinefelter syndrome males may have an organic base for low sex drive and impotence. Half of married couples have an area of sexual incompatibility which may manifest as vague somatic symptoms and general dis-ease.

Sex History Taking: Unique Problems.

Taking a sexual history requires even greater skill than with other systems. Significant obstacles stand between the clinician's capacity to ask a question and the patient's capacity to respond. While comprehensive knowledge is required of the cardiovascular system to cover all the symptom bases, these are typically asked without anxiety or inhibition once the questions are memorized and their rationale understood. Similarly, the patient experiences little or no hesitancy in responding truthfully to the paths of inquiry. Hardly

9

the same exists with sexual history taking. Memorizing a series of questions pertaining to masturbation does not guarantee that the clinician considers the area worthy of time expenditure and hardly eliminates embarrassment when reciting the questions to a middle-aged patient of the opposite sex. Reciprocally, the patient may never have discussed masturbation, may harbor considerable conflict, embarrassment and guilt over the subject, and not see where it is especially relevant to his or her medical history.

An eye-opening exercise in revealing sex history-taking distress is the following: First, choose a medical colleague of the same sex. Ask questions about his or her sexual practices and areas of conflict. Audio record, or better yet, video tape record the interview. Play it back. Listen and watch for hesitancies, vocal tone changes, and facial hints of interviewer distress such as eye contact deflection. Next, role-play a specific sexual problem, for example (if male) a young man with impotency or poor ejaculatory control, or a young father whose child is asking questions about where babies come from. If female, role-play a woman with painful intercourse or a mother whose child asks about babies. Reverse patient-physician roles. Then, choose a colleague of the other sex and repeat. Finally, role-play again, this time as a person of the other sex. This exercise, beyond displaying the unique problems in taking a sex history, is also an effective practice device for learning to interview in specific areas.

The interviewer ill at ease in discussing sexuality communicates a metamessage to the patient which belies the content of the questioning. The metamessage says, "I would really rather *not* hear the answers to your question and hope you have none." Further, the interviewer who conveys a bias regarding the "appropriateness" of certain behaviors shapes patient responses and inhibits elements of patient communication which might elicit physician disapproval.

Sex History Taking: When?

A patient's initial visit prompted by influenza, complicated by otitis media and bronchitis, is hardly the optimal time for a detailed inquiry into sexual attitudes, habits, and possible difficulties. Nor is the appropriate time the third anniversary of the physician-patient relationship. The sexual history should be taken when the initial full medical history is taken. Its inclusion early in the relationship communicates to the patient the physician's appreciation of the importance of sexual health and the physician's comfort in meeting those health needs. Delay in approaching the topic communicates discomfort. The effect when "the subject" is finally broached is comparable to the painfully familiar scene of a father finally initiating discussion of the "facts of life" with his son on his 13th birthday.

Whether or not the initial sexual history elicits significant problem areas may have little primary significance. Perhaps none exist. Perhaps it will take a period of incubation for the patient to experience the necessary degree of trust and comfort to confide a long-standing secret. Or, the early investment may pay off if and when a problem does evolve in a patient who appreciates that the physician is emotionally available for counsel.

Sex History Taking: How?

The opening statement can be, "As I am going to be your physician, I will be responsible for helping maintain your health in all areas. Where your needs may call for more specialized care, I am prepared to refer you to a specialist colleague. One area of health which has been relatively neglected by physicians in the past has been sexual health. It has become increasingly apparent that if we are to fulfill all our responsibilities to patients this important part of our lives must also receive attention. Therefore, I am going to ask you a number of questions in the area of sexuality. Typically, there are certain issues which most frequently raise questions or cause concerns. These include our sexual functioning, the types of sexual experiences we have, our sexual preferences, our sexual adjustment within marriage or outside marriage, the sexual education of our children, the meaning of childhood sex play, teenage sexuality, and so forth. You should know that what we discuss is medically confidential, in the same way as the other areas of your health care." Each interviewer should utilize an opening statement that is personally comfortable. The above has been offered as one model.

An axiom of interviewing style is the "ubiquity" question. Topics are introduced with the assumption that most people have experienced the phenomenon to be introduced. Then the person's own experience in this area is explored. We ask, "*When* or *how* did you first learn about. . ." (rather than "*Did* you learn about. . .?"), "*When* did you first experience. . ." (rather than "*Did* you ever experience. . ."). Or, after the preliminary statement, "Many people experience. . .," the interviewer follows with "What has been your *own* experience with. . .?"

Another axiom is proceeding from less "sensitive" to more "sensitive" areas. Those areas of sexual behavior which are more acceptable and comfortable for discussion are addressed earlier. Topics more likely to elicit anxiety or embarrassment, such as unusual sexual practices, are discussed after greater rapport has been established.

The interviewer's language must be geared to that of the patient. "Fellatio" and "cunnilingus" may be terms familiar to the interviewer and suitable for some patients, whereas "mouth-genital sex," "sucking," "blowing," and "going down" may communicate more effectively with others.

Illustrative Topics

1. *Sexual Dysfunction.* Consider first sexual dysfunction (impotency and premature ejaculation in the male, non-orgasmia or painful intercourse in the female). This topic can be introduced: "Much has been written and discussed during the past few years about sexual incompatibilities within marriage. The work of Masters and Johnson has received much attention with their *successes* (the interviewer promotes optimism) with couples in which the male has difficulty obtaining an erection, or is unable to delay sexual climax, or the female has difficulty in reaching orgasm or has unpleasant intercourse. Most people experience one or more of these difficulties at some time during their sexual relationships. What have your own experiences been?" Or "Most people experience some disappointments, sometimes minor, sometimes major, in the sexual part of their lives. Can you tell me what disappointments you have met?" (No relationship is 100% satisfactory and professional permission to report shortcomings facilitates the revealing of problem areas.) Another facilitating statement is "Frequently, one member of a married couple will desire a variety of sexual activity in which the other person may not be as interested. What has been your own experience in this regard?" (More detailed inquiry in this area is described in Chapter 15.)

2. *Teenage Sexuality.* For parents with teenagers, the history taking can continue: "When children reach teenage, parents typically have new concerns about their child's sexuality. They worry about sexual experimentation, pregnancy, venereal disease, and so on. *Which* of these areas has been of *most* concern to you?"

Education can be an integral part of the interview. "Statistics show us that about one in four girls by the end of high school are engaging in sexual intercourse. Parents then must face the dilemma of teenage pregnancy or contraception. In the past, parents of teenage girls had only limited control (as did their daughters) in preventing unwanted pregnancies. Some parents feel that if they talk with their daughters about pregnancy and perhaps help them with contraceptive control they are endorsing sexual activity (which the parent may find undesirable). Other parents have been impressed by the fact that the vast majority of unwanted teenage pregnancies were the products of intercourse *without* contraception. Clearly the absence of contraception did not *prevent* intercourse, but did have the effect of yielding a more painful consequence. What have been your own views on this?"

Trans-generational differences in sexual values are frequent. Where problems in communication exist between teenager and parent, both generations should be seen separately and then conjointly. "Empathy" statements are useful: "It's often very difficult for those of us who grew up in different generations which held different perspectives on sexuality to feel comfortable with the views of those younger or older." (Then the specific conflict areas are brought into focus.)

Questions and concerns about the physiological changes of puberty are common. They can be acknowledged:

"Many girls growing up receive either no information or hear rumors about the body changes which will occur sometime between 11 and 14. One area in particular is the beginning of monthly bleeding or menstruation. What do you know about what to expect and what this sign of growing up means?" Information provided should stress the unique, positive aspects of becoming a mature woman and the variety in menstrual patterns experienced by young women.

"Many boys during teenage, as their body matures, find that they have dreams with sex in them. They may wake up to find their pajama bottoms wet or that the sheet is wet or stained. They may be confused as to what this means. What has been your experience in this regard?"

3. *The Unmarried Patient Not Living with a Sexual Partner.* The unmarried person's sexuality can be simply explored with this opening statement, "The degree to which unmarried persons have sexual outlets of one or another type varies considerably. Some persons have several partners, others prefer one, others provide themselves release through masturbation, and still others experience no outlet at all. What pattern are you currently following? . . . Has this always been your pattern? . . . Is this your preferred pattern or would you find an alternative preferable? . . . Some unmarried persons find it difficult meeting other persons with whom they might experience a satisfying relationship. To what extent has this been a problem for you?" Then specific questions relating to *sexual dysfunction* can be asked.

4. *Sexual Myths. Seventy* sexual myths and fallacies have been described by McCary (1971). Many plague patients. More common ones may be explored: "Most of us growing up are exposed to many sexual myths or half-

truths which continue to trouble or puzzle us. Are there any which come to mind?" (For males) "One of these are the frequent stories about the importance of penis size. What concerns have you had in this regard?" (For females) "There is much discussion about sexual climax or orgasm. There is talk as to whether women are supposed to have one or several, whether they are supposed to be like inner 'explosions,' whether they are supposed to be 'clitoral' or 'vaginal,' and so on. What questions have you had in this regard?"

5. *Masturbation.* Some interview statements here can be: "Many of us growing up hear a variety of stories about the meaning and implications of masturbation. Some may be upsetting and remain with us well into adulthood. Do you recall when you first learned anything about masturbation? . . . What did you hear? . . . For many of us, these childhood tales continue to exert an influence over us regarding whether we should or should not masturbate. What role do you feel this continues to play in your own life?"

The topic of masturbation is continued if the patient has a child: "Many of us in childhood felt that masturbation was a taboo subject for discussion at home. Most of us practiced it in secret believing our parents would disapprove. Then when we get to be parents ourselves many of us discover that we're not so sure just *how* to best manage these things with our *own* children. What have been your own thoughts on this?"

Again, history taking can also be a time to provide information: "Many parents acknowledge that all children *will* masturbate whether parents like it or not. Therefore, what they decide is to limit it to the private sphere of the child's life in the way that their own adult sexuality is private. Therefore, they do not attempt to prevent masturbation by 'forbidding' it or threatening the child with punishment. Rather they inform the child that it is something to be done alone in the privacy of their room, and not in the classroom, or in the middle of the living room with neighbors visiting." This advice is designed to promote sexual health and reduce conflict within the family regarding an ubiquitous sexual function.

6. *The Homosexual Patient.* If the patient is homosexual, empathy for the uniquely controversial problems of the homosexual can be underscored: "Some say homosexuality is a mental disorder, others an emotional block, others a crime, others a sin. What is your attitude toward your own homosexual orientation? How has the public view of homosexuality affected your own life?" Questioning is designed to find out whether homosexuality is a source of conflict—in the same way that aspects of heterosexuality can be a source of conflict. Keep in mind that homosexuals may have the same sexual dysfunctions as heterosexuals. The interviewer should also know the inci-

dence of homosexuality and treatment results via various approaches for those who wish change (4% of males may be exclusively homosexual, another 6% primarily so; for females the rates appear to be about half (Kinsey *et al.* 1948; 1953); about one-third of highly motivated homosexuals re-orient with psychodynamic or behavioral modification techniques (Bieber *et al.*, 1962; Hatterer, 1970; MacCulloch and Feldman, 1967). (For more detailed patterns of inquiry, see Chapter 5.)

7. *"Unusual" Sex Interests.* "One man's meat is another man's passion." The variety of sexual fantasies may not be finite. Patients can be troubled by their private pornography. Trouble areas can be explored: "Most of us at times experience what we consider to be unusual sexual thoughts, or wish to perform sexual acts which we or others may consider strange. Sometimes we are bothered by these thoughts or impulses. What has been your own experience in this regard?"

8. *Old Age.* Sexual problems during the advanced years result from misinformation or personal mismanagement of various sorts: 1) the false belief that the physiology of old age inevitably leads to radical diminution and cessation of sexual functioning; 2) the misinterpretation of a lessening of sexual drive and incidental sexual dysfunction (*e.g.*, an occasion of male impotency) as the "beginning of the end," with subsequent reluctance to initiate sexual attempts; 3) painful intercourse for the female due to atrophy of the vaginal mucosa and painful uterine contractions during orgasm, secondary to inadequate sex steroid maintenance; and 4) waning physical attractiveness of one or both partners with significant weight gain and poor cosmetic care reducing the sexual interest of the other partner.

Studies of male sexuality in older years indicate that the capacity for erection can be maintained throughout life. Kinsey *et al.* (1948) found that three-quarters of their sample of 70-year old males were potent and that at 75, nearly one-half were still potent. Females in the same age group retain the capacity for multiorgastic response (Masters and Johnson, 1966). For those couples still sexually active at 65, the mean frequency of intercourse has been reported as once per week and at 75, about once per month (Kinsey *et al.*, 1948). Pfeiffer *et al.* (1968) reported that 15% of their sample aged 78 and older were still sexually active.

Some physiological changes do occur with age. For the male the degree of erotic stimulation required for erection becomes greater, the force of ejaculation less, and the refractory period after orgasm, during which the man does not either desire or have the capacity for erection, becomes longer (Masters and Johnson, 1966). For the aging female the length of time required for vaginal lubrication becomes longer and the degree of lubrication less, especially in the sex-steroid starved woman (Masters and Johnson, 1966).

An additional problem for the aging male can be the effects of prostatectomy. Psychological trauma from this procedure can lead to impotency. However, the surgical trauma from transurethral prostatectomy should not affect the capacity for erection. In addition to this reassuring note, the patient should be advised that ejaculation may be retrograde into the bladder, rather than via the penis.

Forearmed with these data and dependent on the circumstances of the patient, questions can be individually tailored and rational counsel provided. With patients in their fifties and beyond, the subject can be approached:

"Many people, as they enter the advanced years in life, believe or are worried that this signals the end of their sex life. Much misinformation has been popularized to perpetuate this myth. What is your understanding about sexuality during the later years? How has the passage of years affected your sexuality?"

9. *Miscellaneous: An Interview Pattern.* "Frequently people have questions about venereal disease (V.D.). What questions do you have?" or

"Frequently people have questions about methods of contraception. What would you like to know about the various methods?" etc.

10. *"Up Front" Sexual Problems.* The above interviewing strategies presume that problems relating to sexuality will be cryptic. What if the "chief complaint" is sexual? In that case general principles of history taking apply. These include the nature and duration of the complaint, the circumstances under which it occurs, and, in the sexual system, the patient's understanding of the cause of the problem and previous efforts at obtaining help. Other chapters in this book dealing with problems of sexual dysfunction, atypical sexual life styles, and sexuality with concurrent medical problems will contribute to the professional's store of knowledge. Having covered the chief complaint, the remainder of the sexual history should not be ignored. Just as the remainder of the health systems are covered when the problem is restricted to one system, inquiry into other areas of sexuality can yield important clues as to how best serve the whole patient.

11. *The Close.* Having exhausted the salient areas of human sexuality, the history taking can be completed: "Is there anything further in the area of sexuality which you would like to bring up *now?* . . . I hope that as questions *do* arise over the course of time we will be able to discuss them here."

Physician Judgmentalism

Our language reveals our personalized attitudes and communicates them to patients. Consider the word "promiscuous" to describe multiple sexual experiences with varied partners. Consider the term "unfaithful" to describe extramarital sexual experiences. In place of moralizing we must be able to integrate and provide objective data regarding what people do and feel, and what evidence exists regarding such experiences. Our language must be nonjudgmental and must permit patients to make decisions based on these facts. The decision must be *theirs*, no matter how repugnant it may be to *our* inner censor.

For a parent who feels masturbation to be a mortal sin, we can only provide a perspective that other equally knowledgeable and well-intentioned parents feel differently. We can point out the data documenting the ubiquity of the behavior and other data associating early-life prohibitions with subsequent sexual inhibitions and dysfunctions. If parents remain adamantly opposed to masturbation, they should state to the child their specific reasons for their opposition. They should assert that it is their religious belief that such behavior is wrong, that not everyone agrees with this belief, and further that masturbation does not cause great harm such as making one go crazy or some other tragic consequence. Parents should realize that the child will know in the course of time the facts about masturbation, and that earlier statements which may frighten the child and are not truthful, may be the basis for later resentment.

For the teenager engaged in repetitive sexual experiences with transient partners, we can counsel on effective methods of contraception and the symptoms and prophylaxis of the venereal diseases. For the adolescent homosexual, we can point out that many homosexuals lead satisfying lives with good emotional and sexual fulfillment but that others are plagued by societal oppression, feel guilty over their orientation, and desire the greater degree of interpersonal stability usually associated with heterosexual marriage and children. We can describe various re-orientation techniques for those who are interested.

It is not easy to be nonjudgmental. Who among us has grown up without strong value feelings about sexual behavior? Many of us are comfortable in what we have settled upon as fitting our life style. Correctness of fit is idiosyncratic. Most of us come from middle-class family systems which may not correspond with our patient's. Were our childhoods uniquely comfortable and sexually *a*conflictual? How many of us had our own sexual questions comfortably answered and did not feel embarrassed talking with our parents about sex? How many of us were not at least temporarily victimized by peer group misinformation and confused by bathroom graffiti and locker-room gossip? Whose parents did not impart their value systems of a generation earlier about masturbation, "sex deviants," intercourse, and marriage. Can we expect these value systems to concur with those of each patient?

Is it our professional responsibility to meet patient needs or our own? Where many medical diseases are concerned, facts abound, and collective research/treatment wisdom and patient-activated guidelines exist. With sexual conduct symptoms of dis-ease exist. The individual who "hurts" because of "too little" sexual conduct or "too much" sexual conduct has a different reason for dis-ease. Our private attitudes may favor the life style of one person over the other; however, that attitude does not belong in the clinical interview or in responsible patient management. It is as inappropriate as if stock ownership in a company producing an orally administered anti-hyper-glycemic drug entered into the decision-making process of carbohydrate regulation in a diabetic. One's private belief about abortion or marital monogamy is irrelevant in meeting the immediate dis-ease of the unmarried teenager or married woman pregnant out-of-wedlock.

Other chapters in this book are intended to provide the clinician with the *facts* upon which to establish *patient-oriented* guidelines for providing clinical help and a data base from which to approach the sexual concerns of patients. When they are read, try again the role-playing exercise of being physician and patient, and adopt problem areas from these topics, be they those of the parents of an intersexed infant or a mentally retarded child, the late pregnancy female, the prematurely ejaculating male, the nonorgasmic female, or the veteran recently paralyzed from the waist down.

Fielding wrote in *Tom Jones,* "Every physician almost hath his favourite disease." Sexual dis-ease will not be each physician's favorite. But, "ease" is as contagious as "dis-ease." Learning to take a sexual history will be both a professional and a personal sexual growth experience. It also carries the potential for "spreading" sexual health.

REFERENCES

Bieber, I. and colleagues. 1962. *Homosexuality: A Psychoanalytic Study.* New York: Basic Books.

Hatterer, L. 1970. *Changing Homosexuality in the Male.* New York: McGraw-Hill.

Kinsey, A., Pomeroy, W., and Martin, C., 1948. *Sexual Behavior in the Human Male.* Philadelphia: Saunders.

Kinsey, A., Pomeroy, W., Martin, C., and Gebhard, P. 1953. *Sexual Behavior in the Human Female.* Philadelphia: Saunders.

MacCulloch, M. and Feldman, M. 1967. Aversion Therapy in Management of Forty-three Homosexuals. Br. Med. J., 2: 594-97.

Masters, W. and Johnson, V. 1966. *Human Sexual Response.* Boston: Little, Brown.

McCary, J. 1971. *Sexual Myths and Fallacies.* Princeton: Van Nostrand and Reinhold.

Pfeiffer, E., Verwoerdt, A., and Wang, H. 1968. Sexual Behavior in Aged Men and Women. Arch. Gen. Psychiat. 19: 753-58.

chapter

3

Anatomy and physiology immerse the beginning health science student. The origins and insertions of myriad muscles, and the devious routes taken by innumerable arteries do not titillate every student. Nor do the mechanisms of sodium and potassium transport during conduction of an action potential necessarily afford a tantalizing introduction to medicine. Yet, anatomy and physiology are basic to understanding bodily functioning. This includes sexual functioning. In contrast to other organ systems, anatomical and physiological studies of human sexuality have only recently been initiated. The human sexual response cycle and notably the female response was first detailed in the 1960's. The findings of basic science have clinical implications. We address that interface.

Editor

Sexual Anatomy and Physiology: Clinical Aspects

MILTON DIAMOND, Ph.D

Classically, anatomy and physiology are two of the prime basic sciences upon which clinical practice depends. This is equally true for sexual matters as well as for other medical areas, yet regrettably, most anatomical relationships and physiological processes associated with sex are not made clear to the student. This is unfortunate since it takes no training for a person to be aware of his or her body and its functioning, and all patients have many ideas of what is normal or expected, even if quite mistaken.

This chapter will attempt to examine and make clear the most pertinent relations of basic anatomy and physiology to clinical practice. Those psychological parameters associated with the anatomical and physiological factors discussed will also be included. This is a sharp departure form typical anatomy and physiology presentations but clinically is crucial. Penis size, for example, while anatomically and physiologically of no more consequence than foot size, for most adult men, looms psychologically much larger and more important. With this in mind, even if the subject is not brought up by the patient, the wise physician will often take the initiative in discussing many of these topics with a patient in the course of a physical examination or whenever appropriate. This will remove the onus and embarrassment from the patient. It may in some cases also be wise to discuss the matter with a spouse or parents since they, too, may share concerns similar to the patient's.

ANATOMY

Clinical problems of sexual anatomy most generally involve false expectations about what is normal. To a lesser degree, they are developmental prob-

21

lems. Some of the latter problems will require and be amenable to therapeutic treatment, either surgical or medical; regrettably many won't. Most problems and concerns about what is normal, fortunately, can be handled by cogent and sympathetic counseling.

Normal Development. Deeply engraved by culture and tradition, everyone develops with an image of what is desired in body shape and capacity. The tall, dark, and handsome stereotype for males is well known as is the female counterpart of the long-legged, large-breasted, and wasp-waisted beauty. Most often an individual accepts nature's decree which rarely fits the stereotype. However, concern may be experienced, for example, with being over- or underweight, too short if male, too tall if female, or having acne. These may reflect on an individual's self-appraisal of sexual identity and body image. These are all readily obvious public manifestations and are taken as reflections of an individual's masculinity and femininity.

There is no known correlation of body configuration and sexual capability. Being tall or short, fat or slim, or having a large or small penis, or large or small breasts, does not of itself confer any particular type of concomitant sexual functioning. Psychologically, however, there may be, in individual cases, a strong correlation between anatomy and ability. A male with a small penis or a female with small breasts may have a severe reluctance to undress or project sexually; and the prospect of coitus may frighten such individuals, primarily because it threatens exposure. On the other hand, an individual whose genitals are obviously large may have an exaggerated view of their importance.

The Male. Aside from general body and face configuration, most men are concerned with penis size. With a wide degree of variation, the average adult penis, when measured from the pubic symphysis to the meatus, ranges from 8.5 to 10.5 cm. in length and 2.5 to 3.5 cm. in diameter when flaccid to about double that in length when erect—15.0 ± 2.5 cm. There is a slight increase of about 0.5 cm. in diameter with erection. The size of a man's penis is not related to other aspects of body build and is not predictable by race or affected by ethnicity, sexual experience, or masturbation.

Male patients will believe many myths about penises. Two of the more common myths are that a large penis is more satisfying to a woman, and a circumcised penis is more sensitive and therefore more liable to premature ejaculation. There is no evidence for either belief. Significantly, while a small penis conceptually disturbs most men, a large penis may conceptually disturb many women; they fear their inability to accommodate. Men are seldom concerned with their scrotum or other parts of their external anatomy. They are, however, concerned with their testes and ability to function, both sexually and reproductively, should any medical concern involve their urogenital system. Two common concerns involve sequelae to venereal disease and vasectomy. It behooves the attending physician to assure and reassure the patient that urogenital diseases, when adequately treated, and vasectomy, when properly done, will leave no deleterious occult effects. Typically any positive sexual capabilities present prior to the treatment or surgery will remain afterward.

Three developmental problems of males, sure to arouse concern, are cryptorchidism, hypospadias, and epispadias. Since these problems are discernible at birth, these are to be discussed with the parents since they will soon be aware of the abnormality. The manifestations of ambiguous genitalia call for all cases of cryptorchidism and hypo- or epispadias to be examined for evidence of intersexuality or adrenal hyperplasia (Diamond, 1965; 1968).

While the testes usually descend to the scrotum sometime after the seventh fetal month, approximately 5% of males retain undescended or abdominal testis at birth. The unexplained absence of a testis for the parents or individual may be psychologically traumatic and should be attended to medically and with counseling. For the majority of these males, descent will occur with subsequent differential growth of the body, suspensory ligament of the testis, and gubernaculum. When descent is inordinately delayed, chorionic gonadotropins have been found to be of value. When hormone therapy fails, surgery is called for. If this is prolonged, sterility *may* result; also, the incidence of malignancy is higher in abdominal testes.

Hypospadias and epispadias occur in females as well as males but are of importance in the female only if related to incontinence (Anhalt and Carlton, 1973). In the male, these are problems of functional and psychological consequence. Hypospadias is much more common than epispadias and, as a genetic trait, tends to manifest itself along family lines. Aside from the obvious problem with an unfused urethral groove, most often, is the more difficult problem of a rudimentary scarred corpus spongiosum which forms a chordee, causing the penis to curve ventrally. This may make erection difficult and typical intercourse impossible. Cosmetic and functional correction of the hypospadiac condition is most often possible and should be recommended. In all cases, psychological counseling should be part of the treatment since, post-surgically, many men still abstain from sexual contact (Farkas and Hynie, 1970).

The Female. Women have their own concerns with body image. Most commonly, they worry about weight distribution, mainly over their hips and thighs. Regarding their sexual organs, a recent survey found approximately 25% of the female respondents dissatisfied with their breasts and 9% very dissatisfied (Berscheid et al., 1973). In regard to breasts, it is both shape as well as size which can arouse concern. Most often women complain of breasts they think are small. The breast size desired is, in contrast to penis size, not abstractly large but rather proportionate to body size. As with male anatomy, there is no known correlation of body configuration and sexual ability or femininity except as psychologically perceived by the individuals involved within culturally fostered stereotypes.

Micromastia is most often developmental. It may, however, occasionally be acquired as via postpartum loss of breast tissue. Often the flat-chested women will herself have tried to build up her breasts with exercises and hormone creams. The endocrine treatments, particularly high estrogen and progesterone, may work if the etiology of the problem is hypogonadal, but, in an otherwise normal woman, is without much effect.

Macromastia is less often the object of professional or lay conversation or folklore, yet it is probably a much more serious medical problem. Overly large breasts, (an issue of particular sensitivity among pubescent and teenage girls), aside from being objects of ridicule, may be physical burdens to bear due to poorly distributed weight and the impingement or stress on thoracic nerve and vascular roots. For example, motor and sensory processes associated with ulnar distribution have been compromised. Women complain of back and neck pains. Chronic pulmonary or cardiac diseases may be significantly affected by macromastia (Kaye, 1973).

In men, gynecomastia often accompanies liver diseases and alcoholism. This quite often becomes of sufficient size to be the presenting complaint. After attending to the underlying etiology, cosmetic removal of the excess breast tissue is possible.

Two breast conditions which are seen often enough to warrant comment are bilateral asymmetry and inverted nipples. Both are developmental, and most often require only counseling and reassurance to the woman. She may deal cosmetically with the asymmetry, and the nipple inversion will not hinder her ability to nurse.

Most women have never closely inspected their vagina. This is in contrast with adolescent males where comparison with others and inspection of self are common. This lack of self-inspection, along with standard misinformation leads many women to welcome offered information. In contrast with men, many women are apprehensive about a large penis. It is not appreciated that the vagina is a highly distendable yet adaptive organ which presents only a potential space, not an actual one. The penis acts as an appropriate dilator, bringing the vagina to conformational shape. As with all biological phenomena, however, there are extremes in size. An overly large (considered in diameter) vagina is acquired usually from stretching at parturition. Short or overly tight vaginas are usually developmental. Since genital shape varies with physiological state, a diagnosis of a small vagina must be made when the woman is in a plateau stage (see below) of sexual response. The vagina, from an average resting size of about 8 cm. in depth for a nullipara, distends and elongates with increase in sexual stimulation. The amount of elongation depends on the extent of dilation. Quite often with advanced age and sexual abstinence, secondary stenosis may occur. Here adequate hormone therapy and repeated sexual stimulation and coitus often can ameliorate the problem.

Within the vagina, some women report areas which are particularly responsive to stimuli, so-called centers of sexual sensory perception. These are located along the vaginal walls at approximately the 4:00 and 8:00 o'clock areas approximately two-finger joints inside the introitus.

Some women voice concern over "being too loose," "not feeling the penis," or will give some other indication of a vagina-related problem. Often, these concerns can be ameliorated by a combination of counseling and exercises. Helpful exercises, first promulgated for urinary stress—incontinence, involve strengthening of the pubococcygeus muscle as well as the pelvic diaphragm. Generally, this involves the woman alternately contracting and expanding those muscles she can identify as necessary to control her urinary flow or childbirth process. Daily routine sets of contractive exercises have proven helpful, regardless of the particular tone in the vaginal muscle, in assisting women toward a positive view of their vaginal sensations and responses (Kegel, 1952). These exercises quite often help a woman increase her satisfaction and pleasure from coitus.

It had been, for some time, a medical misconception that vaginal lubrication was due to secretions emanating from glandular tissue of the uterine cervix. Indeed, such uterine secretions are perfuse but clinically limited to the mucus plug for the cervical outlet. In contrast, the vagina is without such obvious secretory tissue. Vaginal lubrication is due to a sweating-like phenomenon of the vaginal walls. As penile erection signals sexual arousal and excitement in the male, the wall of the vaginal barrel becomes lined with a transudation-like mucoid material. This material quickly provides evidence of the female's sexual arousal and lubrication for coition. (For most women, therefore, if sufficiently aroused, artificial lubricants are not usually needed.)

Both men and women often harbor fallacies about the hymen. These fallacies may have significant cultural ramifications where women must or choose to demonstrate anatomical virginity. The hymen remains as the demarcation of the developmental dual origin of the vaginal barrel from the distal portion of the medullary ducts and proximal portion of the vaginal vestibule as an invagination of the urogenital sinus. With this origin, its shape and structure is quite variable, ranging from almost nonexistent to imperforate.

The hymen may exist intact as a covering for the vaginal orifice until coitus, or it may be broken or pierced by accident or experimentation. Most hymens prior to coitus will allow passage of a vaginal tampon or inspecting finger. Some will stretch quite easily. However, a hymen also may be of such firm consistency as to defy penile penetration. In such cases, after consultation with the woman involved, self-regulated dilation of the hymen at home is possible. In more obstinate cases, cutting the hymen in a simple office procedure will prevent unneeded frustration at the time of first intercourse. Virginity as a hymenal counterpart is one thing and, as a state of mind or body, is something else. A woman may have had quite a variety of sexual experiences and yet come to delivery with an incompletely perforated hymen. Virgins, on the other hand, may have only small hymenal remnants in evidence at the time of their first intercourse. Reconstruction of the hymen is not feasible, but a simple tenuously placed suture across a side of the hymenal ring most often will serve the intended social purpose.

Both your male and female patients would welcome factual information about the clitoris due to its prominence in folklore and many marriage manuals. Most women have never seen their own clitoris and most men are hesitant to admit their ignorance of it. It would be wise during a physical examination to show your female patients (and quite often their spouses), with the use of mirrors, their clitoris, and general peroneal anatomy. Despite the homology with the penis, the clitoris in most women is quite small but variable in size and does not get erect. With sexual excitement, it will become engorged and will increase in sensitivity, however, Also, in comparison with the penis, which for most males is the prime focus for erotic sensation, during masturbation or coitus, the clitoris may or may not be the focus for the female. The glans clitoris contains the highest density of Pacinian pressure receptors in the body, yet most women do not masturbate with direct clitoral stimulation nor does direct contact occur during coitus. Stretching and pressure of the mons and labia transfer erotic stimuli sufficient for erotic sensation. Some women, however, do desire direct clitoral stimulation; and each woman should choose and indicate to her partner what is most desirable.

Comments about two more areas of anatomy should prove helpful in understanding some common sexual practices and attitudes. The first concerns a general reminder that the sensory distribution of the pudendal nerves includes rami from the dorsal nerve of the penis or clitoris, the perineal nerve, and the inferior rectal nerve. These three rami coverage to terminate on common sacral segments S-2, S-3, and S-4, but mostly S-3. Thus, for some individuals, sensations received from the anus, labia, scrotum, penis, or clitoris are interpreted as similarly pleasurable (Diamond, 1972). Cultural ramifications will influence the way an individual uses this sensory capacity. While anal intercourse for men and women is one example of how these sensations may reflect a pleasurable focus, so is the finding that some women masturbate or increase their sensate focus by gluteal or thigh activity.

The second area for comment is in regard to body effluents. In the process of general sexual counseling, I have found it helpful to point out that males and females have different approaches to their body fluids. Consider that the typical male has been ejaculating and the normal female has been menstruating since puberty. By the age of 18, then, the male has about 4 or 5 years of experience dealing routinely with semen and the female similarly has about 6 or 7 years experience dealing with menstrual blood. Each person routinely, after several exposures, becomes accustomed to his or her body products. For each, however, at the time of encountering the other sex's effluents, distaste and repugnance are often felt and expressed. Counseling as to the analogous, naturalness, and relative feelings of each sex to these fluids generally eases the situation. Analogously, both men and women often are relieved to learn that urine is sterile and does not come from the vaginal orifice but from the urethral opening on the floor of the vaginal vestibule.

PHYSIOLOGY

The physiological processes attendant to sexual expression are in some ways similar to those for any behavior, yet in many ways are unique. Any sexual behavior might be considered to comprise, in some degree, the individual being in a sexual state involving what I term an *Aspect, Phase,* and *Mechanism* (Table 1). The understanding of the components of this state is crucial for any clinical evaluation of sexual expression, since every problem involves some actual or believed incoordination or malfunction of these components. Just as any adequate treatment requires accurate diagnosis in dealing with sexual concerns, one must first be able to diagnose which components are affected before treatment can begin.

Aspects.

Typically, a sexual process is comprised of both of two aspects: psychological and somatic. A psychological aspect might be, but is not necessarily, psychogenic. It may remain psychic or become somatic. No body or genital response need be apparent in pure psychic behavior. For example, pornography or fantasy may be evaluated for sexual content on a psychic level. Via cognitive processes of either learned or innate origin, pornography or fantasy may or may not be arousing. The same might be said of any thought of sexual nature. The present discussion of physiological processes is an example of a mental aspect of sex which is usually nonarousing. In contrast, the fantasies typically associated with masturbation or coitus are mental *and* arousing.

We might distinguish between psychological processes which are either cognitive or instinctive. For the present discussion, a sharp definition of instinctive is not held to. Here, I am only trying to distinguish between a thought process, which is knowingly, willfully, and consciously called forth by the individual (cognitive) from one which is not (instinctive). Instinctive mental processes are less easy to define but are exemplified by those thoughts or deeds which seem reflexive or automatic. These instinctive thoughts may or may not be erotic. An individual who passes an open window and glancingly sees a nude in the room and turns with a double-take to look again may view the person inside with erotic or nonerotic interest. The turn to look again at a nude body may be considered reflexive.

In contrast to psychological aspects are those body responses entailed under the heading of somatic aspects. A penile erection, for example, if engendered by stimuli from the urinary bladder, is phenotypically a peripheral sexual expression. It is usually not construed as sexual. The erection, however, may engender cognitive sexual aspects. Similarly, priapism is a penile erection without sexual content. In contrast, an erect penis used in coitus is a peripheral, erotic manifestation due to situational and appropriate sexual content.

Before proceeding, consider these clinical cases where the concordance of cephalic and peripheral aspects of sexual expression are at issue. These should help understand why the diagnostic distinction is made.

Case 1. A 26-year-old male in bed with his wife cannot get an erection on their wedding night.

Psychologically, the situation is cognitively arousing and instinctively erotic. In contrast, peripherally and somatically (judging from his penis), the individual is phenotypically not aroused. How he further behaves may be construed as situationally non-erotic or erotic.

Case 2. A 39-year-old woman complains that, although she engages in intercourse with adequate vaginal lubrication, she does not enjoy it and does not reach orgasm.

Psychologically, she is not cognitively aroused nor is she demonstrating instinctive eroticism. Somatically, she is behaving as if aroused and situationally erotic.

Obviously, when both cephalic and somatic aspects are in concert, we can say the individual exhibits sexual health. When there is involuntary discordance between cephalic and somatic aspects, we can consider the individual in ill health.

Phases.

The work of Masters and Johnson (1966; 1970) has brought a good deal of attention to what has been termed the Sex Response Cycle. This cycle refers to progressive, recordable anatomical and physiological changes which typically accompany somatic genital sexual expression.

The response cycle may be arbitrarily considered to have six phases, each with concomitant cephalic and peripheral aspects: resting, excitement, plateau, orgasmic, postorgasmic, and resolution.* For outline-organizational purpose, these phases will be discussed briefly, then enlarged upon.

Most often, an individual will be sexually at rest. While at rest, psychologically and somatically, the individual will be in a nonsexual state attending to other matters or a subconscious state receptive to sexual stimuli. As sexual interest develops, either due to psychogenic or peripheral stimuli, the individual enters into the excitement phase. This is marked, in both men and women, by a progressive increase in vasocongestion and muscular tension—primarily in the genitals. Vasocongestion and muscular tension are both signs of somatic sexual response. Most commonly, this is evidenced by penile erection in the male and vaginal lubrication in the female. It is not always easy to ascertain what it is that initiates sexual excitement. While it may be psychogenic or somatogenic in origin, its continuation generally depends upon both cognitive and situational reinforcement.

The excitement phase continues to increase in intensity into a plateau phase when the period of vasocongestion and muscular tension levels off and

---

* Masters and Johnson consider four parts to the cycle. I have added consideration of *resting* and *postorgasmic* phases.

a high state of sexual interest is maintained. The duration of the plateau phase is indefinite, short or long, and limited by the effectiveness of the cognitive and situational stimuli and the desire, training, and biology of the individuals involved. It is from this phase that an individual can shift to orgasm.

The orgasmic phase is relatively brief and marked by a rapid release from the developed vasocongestion and myotonia. The onset of orgasm may be both psychogenically and somatically fostered with any site in focus. Its primary site of appreciation is cephalic while its primary site of release is pelvic. Primarily, it is the penis, prostate, and seminal vesicles in the male, and the clitoris, vagina, and uterus in the female which are involved. The orgasmic release, coming after a period of sexual tension, is distinct and has been thus termed "climax" in recognition of its peak psychological and physical intensity and attendent feeling of satisfaction. For men, this is typically, but not obligatorily, accompanied by ejaculation. In women, despite myths to the contrary, ejaculation cannot occur. Copious secretions and transudate may, however, flow.

Following orgasm, the subsequent postorgasmic phase may be quite different for men and women. In general, the male will be found to be relatively refractory to further sexual stimuli. His penis will detumesce and he will pass through a resolution phase and return to a relaxed *resting* phase. This will be sleep in many cases. The transition will involve a reversal of the reactions that occurred during plateau and excitement phases. Peripherally, a generalized decrease in vasocongestion and myotonia will occur and psychologically, a decrease in arousal will be noted. While females too may quickly resolve toward sleep, it is common for many, however, to remain responsive to sexual stimulation. A postorgasmic refractory phase would be, for them, unusual. They might return to a plateau stage from which they invite additional stimulation to return to an additional subsequent orgasm. Following satisfaction, a resolution phase follows for both males and females. Resolution might be considered involutional and recuperative.

Concomitant with these phases are genital and extragenital responses which are typical for men and women. In men, the most noted changes are those that occur in the penis and scrotum. For women, changes occur in breasts and pudenda.

Men in general show greater consistency from one to another and from one time to another in their response cycle. Women, in contrast, seem much more variable and labile. For some women, excitement proceeds quickly through plateau to orgasm and orgasm is explosive, accompanied by a great display of involuntary movement and vocalization. For other women, the cycle is relatively slow in building, controlled in amplitude, and long lasting. For a minority of women, orgasm never occurs; for many it is intermittently absent. Any one woman may, at different times, display a different pattern. Men, except during old age or sickness, rarely are consistently without orgasm.

Orgasm is the "final common path" for physiological release from the built-up mental and muscular tension. The inputs to this release are individually variable and distinctions between various input sites (*e.g.* clitoris or vagina) are not necessarily crucial and often specious. For orgasm, the somatic sensate focus may be from the penis or scrotum in the male and from the vagina, breast, or clitoris in the female. The psychological aspect of coitus may involve concentration on the present partner or act, or fantasy about other times and persons. While physiologically an orgasm may be quite variable in intensity, attention to these peripheral aspects is less crucial than attention to the psychological aspects of satisfaction. Satisfaction for both men and women may be had *without* orgasm. The satisfaction of the individuals involved should be the primary concern of the partners and physician rather than a focus on presence or intensity of orgasm (Fink *et al.*. 1973).

The concept of simultaneous orgasm deserves comment. For some couples, this is a positive objective which demands attainment and its absence is viewed as a sign of sexual incompatibility. For other couples, it is of no consequence or an obstacle to satisfaction. Consider some relative advantages and disadvantages of each and see how in this matter, as in most other sexual matters; the rule "to each his/her own" prevails.

Simultaneous orgasm is viewed positively by those who consider coital activity an endeavor in which the couple attempts to demonstrate the ability to pleasure each other in a parallel manner. They consider the parallel progression of sexual excitement to orgasm and resolution as providing the greatest degree of satisfaction.

Others consider most satisfying those activities which allow each to benefit from the activities found most pleasurable without regard to parallelism. For example, one partner may enjoy a long excitement phase or being maintained at a plateau level while another may desire a rapid orgasm and maintained postorgasmic resolution phase. During orgasm, most women desire deep vaginal penetration and continual and sustained direct or indirect clitoral stimulation. By contrast, males at orgasm tend to withdraw their pelvis and halt thrusting movements. These processes seem mutually conflicting. Thus satisfaction may be attained by nonsimultaneous orgasm since each partner can attend to the pleasuring needs of the other. The psychological aspects of sex allow for satisfaction to be derived from receiving release from one's own sexual tensions or giving release to another. For many individuals the subjective feeling of close personal warmth and body contact is more satisfying than the orgastic pleasure *per se.*

SEXUAL MECHANISMS

It is advantageous to consider physical sexual expression as dependent upon three categories of sexual mechanisms. The neural tissues and physiological aspects involved are not necessarily separate for each, but each has its own measurable and clinically pertinent characteristics. Overlap and simultaneous functioning of these mechanisms may or may not occur. The three mechanisms involved are: *arousal mechanisms, copulatory mechanisms,* and *orgastic mechanisms* (Table 1).

Arousal mechanisms are associated with those sensory processes involved in receiving and interpreting sexual clues. Examples are visual, tactile, auditory, and olfactory stimuli which interact centrally to transform the in-

TABLE 1
Outline for the physiology of sexual behavior

I. Aspects
    Psychological
        Cognitive: nonarousing; arousing
        Instinctive or reflexive: nonerotic; erotic
    Somatic
        Phenotypic
        Situational or experiential

II. Phases
    Resting
    Excitement
    Plateau
    Orgasmic
    Postorgasmic
    Resolution

III. Mechanisms
    Arousal mechanisms   Erection mechanisms
    Copulatory mechanisms   involve   Lubricating mechanisms
    Orgastic mechanisms   Sensory modalities
                                              Hormonal balance
                                            Neuromuscular diasthesis

All are biologically structured and environmentally mediated.

dividual from a resting phase to excitement and through plateau and orgasm (*cf.* Diamond *et al.*, 1972).

Copulatory mechanisms are those physiological processes associated with genital sexual expressions. These include, for example, penile and nipple erection and vaginal lubrication. Orgastic mechanisms associated with orgasm include, in the male, ejaculatory processes, and in the female, perhaps vocalization processes.

Thresholds for responses by all three sets of mechanisms, as well as the above-mentioned aspects and phases, are dependent upon genetics, inherent neural bias, endocrine levels, and receptor tendencies. Also interacting are cultural alterations to biology via learning and conditioning. Typically, these processes have sex distinctions. For example, visual arousal sensitivities may differ for men and women (Diamond *et al.*, 1972) or the orgastic mechanisms of females may be programmed for multiple and repeated response while this is rarely so for males except when they are young. The biases placed upon these processes (aspects, phases, and mechanisms) are most crucially diasthetic but subject to postnatal mediation (Diamond, 1965; 1968; 1975). The organization for these diasthetic influences is genetic and endocrine in origin; the activation of the influences is maturational and environmental. Thus, just as anatomical problem situations may be developmental or acquired, so may be physiological ones. It should further be kept in mind that, as in the other physiological processes, these sexual mechanisms are subject to biochemical influences. Thus, many drugs as well as steroid and other hormone levels can significantly mediate sexual expression. For example, administered androgens typically increase libidinal intensity in females and administered estrogens or progesterone decrease libido in males. Other side effects of steroids are common. All neurological problems must, until proven otherwise, be suspect as having concomitant effects on some aspects of sexual expression.

Diagnostically, it is crucial to determine whether a mechanism has never been manifest (a primary condition) or has been lost subsequently (a secondary condition). For example, a male who never had an erection would be diagnosed as having a primary impotence. An individual who does not have an erection with a certain partner or at certain times would be diagnosed as having a secondary impotence. A primary loss would tend to indicate a developmental problem in comparison to a secondary loss, which would indicate an acquired or situational difficulty. Appropriate treatment is predicated on making such diagnostic distinctions (Weiss *et al.*, 1973).

Anatomically, problems are first best analyzed as to whether they are developmental or acquired, and actual or imagined. Physiologically, the situation is more complex. A situation or function will have psychological as well as somatic aspects and be related to various sexual phases and mechanisms. All features must be considered for effective diagnosis and treatment.

Most commonly, a patient's presenting sexual complaint will involve some conceived or actual anatomical or physiological disorder or problem. While both anatomy and physiology are basic medical sciences, their sexual aspects are rarely taught. This chapter hopefully affords a means of dealing with the most frequent of such concerns and problems and also provides a framework from which others can be appraised and managed.

REFERENCES

Anhalt, M. A. and Carlton, C. E., Jr. 1973. Hypospadias and Epispadias, Med. Aspects Human Sex 7: 218-226.

Berscheid, E., Walsten E., and Bohrnstedt, G. 1973. The Happy American Body. A Survey Report. Psychol. Today 7: 119.

Diamond, M. 1965. A Critical Evaluation of the Ontogeny of Human Sexual Behavior. Quart. Rev. Biol. 40: 147-75.

Diamond, M. 1968. Genetic-endocrine Interactions and Human Psychosexuality. In *Perspectives in Reproduction and Sexual Behavior*. (M. Diamond, ed.) 417-443. Bloomington: Indiana Univ. Press.

Diamond, M. 1972. Anal Eroticism. Med. Aspects Human Sex 6: 178.

Diamond, M., Diamond, A. L., Mast, M. 1972, Visual Sensitivity and Sexual Arousal Levels during the Menstrual Cycle. J. Nerv. Ment. Dis. 155: 170-176.

Diamond, M. (In press). Human Sexual Development. In *Human Sexuality*. (F. A. Beach, ed.) New York: McGraw-Hill.

Farkas, L. G. and Hynie, J. 1970. After-effects of Hypospadias Repair in Childhood. Postgrad. Med. 47: 103.

Fink, P. J., Murphy, R., Murphy J., Fisher, S. de Moya, A., de Moya, D. Diamond, M. and Gray, M. 1973. What is the Basis for the Distinction Many Patients make between Vaginal and Clitoral Orgasms? Med. Aspects Human Sex 7: 84.

Kaye, B. L. 1973. Micromastia vs Macromastia. Med. Aspects Human Sex 7: 96-123.

Kegel, A. H. 1952. Sexual Functions of the Pubococcygeus Muscle. West. J. Obstet.-Gynecol. 60: 521.

Masters, W. H. and Johnson, V. E. 1966. *Human Sexual Response*. Boston: Little, Brown.

Masters, W. H. and Johnson, V. E. 1970. *Human Sexual Inadequacy*. Boston: Little, Brown.

Weiss, H. D., Diamond, M., and Gergen, J. A. 1973. Mechanism of Erection. Med. Aspects Human Sex 7: 28.

chapter

4

Is there a "sexual revolution"? Are the rates of premarital and extramarital sexuality undergoing dramatic change? Are sexual practices affected by social class? Is male and female sexuality changing differentially? Has the availability of female contraceptive devices had a dramatic impact on the sexuality of adolescent patients? What do most people do sexually, before, in place of, or during marriage? Why is this information important for the physician?

Most of us tend to generalize about the remainder of the population from our own sexual experiences. Most of us grow up with relatively clear ideas of what constitutes appropriate sexual conduct between males and females. Each of us, physician and patient, has our personal sexual value system. At the junction of physician attitudes and patient behavior, the medical interests of the patient can be compromised.

Each patient's sexuality is unique. Awareness of the varieties of contemporary sexual behavior, and its place within a cultural perspective, can cast both the physician's and the patient's behavior against the broader sexual landscape. Hopefully, this perspective will reduce not only the potential for contaminating the patient's sexuality with our own but also any attempt to graft onto the patient our own personalized value system.

Editor

Heterosexual Relationships of Patients: Premarital, Marital, and Extramarital

IRA L. REISS, Ph.D.

One key service that sociology can provide for the physician in the area of sex is to help free him or her from the many social myths that prevail regarding sexual relationships. Most areas of human behavior develop belief systems that are infused with erroneous ideas. Sex is an area where emotion runs high and one would expect many myths to prevail. Sociology can provide a more objective perspective on human sexuality and act as a corrective on such myths.

The 19th century approach to human sexuality in the Western world was heavily moralistic. Medical doctors such as Acton and Brown were putting forth the idea that "normal" women were not sexually active and if a woman was that way, her clitoris could be removed to correct that "abnormality" (Comfort, 1967). Masturbation was often medically viewed as "abnormal." The psychiatric approach of Kraft-Ebbing, Havelock Ellis, and others was heavily oriented to "disturbed" and "abnormal" aspects (Krich, 1963). Commonly used terms were expressions with strong moral implications such as "proper" sexual behavior, "natural" tendencies, and such. An objective, scientific, research approach to human sexuality was not present in the 19th century, except in small and very mild doses.

The 20th century witnessed the rise of social science but in the area of human sexuality scientific objectivity was often sacrificed to personal moral judgments. Most of the writings on human sexuality chose to emphasize particular moral points like the value of virginity rather than to report findings on causes and consequences of different sexual practices. The college

37

courses on marriage that began in the 1920's were also moralistic and applied, rather than scientific and research oriented. Such courses became, in many colleges, little more than "advice to the lovelorn" courses and were of little scholarly value.

It was the advent of the World War II that signaled the rapid rise of the social sciences. The army found social science to be of value in measuring the attitudes of soldiers toward racial integration of their units and in the study of reasons for high or low troop morale. At the end of the war, scientific, sociological surveys were the basis for the point system on which soldiers were discharged. These experiences with the potential worth of social science research led to federal funds being set aside for studies of human relationships. The end result was great encouragement of scientific research in all areas including the sexual. Almost all of the valuable scientific work on human sexuality has been published in the three decades following World War II.

THE VIRGINITY MYTH

One popular myth that is still believed by many is that in the Victorian era and the Puritan period, we had a nation of people who were largely virginal before marriage. The historical evidence argues otherwise. Two hundred years ago, in Groton, Massachusetts, we have church records indicating that one of every three brides confessed fornication to her minister (Calhoun, 1945). Such confessions were typically made only by females who were pregnant and thus the proportion of nonvirginal females was probably even higher.

Similar evidence exists for the Victorian era in the late 19th century. It seems that open prostitution was widespread at that time and under the counter hard core pornography was available in most major cities (Winick and Kinsie, 1971). There likely was a higher percentage of female virgins than today but still many females were experienced (Kinsey estimated about one in every four females in his sample, born before 1900, was nonvirginal). Males have always had the vast majority experienced in coitus before adulthood and the 19th century was no exception. In fact there is no society in the world where the majority of males remain virginal even to the end of their teens. Thus, the evidence, briefly examined above, indicates that there never was a time when all men and women were virginal before marriage.

What is the importance of this knowledge to the physician? First, it affords the doctor perspective on patients who may come in with guilt feelings regarding sexual behavior. The doctor with this historical knowledge is aware that sexual experience has always been widespread but, despite that fact, there has been opposition to such freedom by the church and by many parents. The doctor will recognize more easily the cause of the patient's dilemma when realizing that most of us internalize the historical feelings of wrongness of sex outside of marriage but *also* internalize the peer group support and the free courtship system that promotes sexual opportunity.

Another benefit of this historical perspective to the doctor is the deeper understanding of male-female differences and similarities in sexuality. I mentioned above that male sexual permissiveness has always been very high but female permissiveness varied more over time and place. Because of the emphasis in medical education on physiology, we are likely to believe that male-female differences in sexual outlook and performance are physiologically based. Without getting involved in the many aspects of such a question, our observation is that the percentage of women who rarely or never have orgasm has dramatically reduced from 28% to 15% in the last 30 years (Hunt, 1973) and the percentage of women engaging in premarital intercourse has risen from 25% in 1900 to 75% in 1973. Regional differences have also been found. Reiss (1967) reported that California women were more sexually permissive than New York women. Finally, Hunt reported in 1973 that 25% of married women under 35 had experienced anal intercourse whereas in the 1940's this was a very rare practice. Female sexuality has changed more than male sexuality. This is probably due to the fact that males have been in power and thus are unlikely to restrict their own sexual permissiveness. By contrast with our own, many cultures in Polynesia have sexual equality before marriage (Malinowski, 1929).

The physician knowing this equality potential will be prepared to meet a wide range of reported female sexual responsiveness and will be aware that female responsiveness can be altered if one desires. By removing the belief that females are inevitably less sensuous than males, the doctor opens up a wide variety of alternative treatments that otherwise would not be considered or discussed. Whatever physiological or anatomical differences exist between the sexes, cultural training can lead to sexual equality between males and females. In fact, the Masters and Johnson (1966) data indicate that females are more capable of multiple orgasms than males. There is a real doubt that males could be trained to equal the high rate of multiple orgasm of such women. Thus, there is little evidence to establish an immutable male sexual superiority.

PLATEAUS AND PEAKS IN THE 20th CENTURY

A second popular myth about sexuality asserts that increased sexual permissiveness has occurred consistently over the decades of this century. The evidence from national studies by Kinsey *et al* (1948, 1953), Klassen *et al*. (1972), Simon and Gagnon (1974), Reiss (1967), and Zelnik and Kantner (1972) is among the best available for examining trends. Hunt's recent data (1973) are also relevant. Studies of more limited samples of college students are also available (Bell, 1970; Christensen, 1970; and Ehrman, 1959). The picture that emerges is one of dramatic changes in our sexual lives occurring in two very short periods of this century, with the intervening decades acting as time for consolidation of radical changes. These two periods of rapid change are: 1) 1915 to 1920 and 2) 1965 to 1970. While these time periods are really estimates, the data indicate that premarital non-virginity rates of females doubled in the first period from 25% to 50% and in the second period rose to about 75%. Marital orgasm rates for females also rose noticeably during both periods. In the first period, extramarital coital rates rose to 50% of the husbands and 30% of the wives having one extramarital affair by age 40 (Kinsey *et al*. 1953). Evidence from Hunt indicates that most of the increase in the recent period in extramarital coitus is for females under the age of 25. Guilt may accompany innovative sexual behavior. One way of overcoming guilt is repetition of the sexual behavior that first aroused the guilt. Reiss (1967) reported that the vast majority of females who experienced guilt repeated the behavior until they eventually came to accept it.

These two periods were times of basic social change outside of the sexual sphere as well (O'Neill, 1967). The 1915 to 1920 period was the entry of America as a world power—a time when the U. S. had entered fully into the life style of an industrial society. By the 1965 to 1970 period America had become what is popularly called a post-industrial society. That term refers to a society that has focused its attention less on production of goods and services and more on the fair and equitable distribution of those goods and services. Civil rights legislation, women's rights, and other minority group movements all evidenced this change.

Another index of rapid social change is the presence of a major world war in both periods. In the earlier period it was World War I and in the recent period it was the Vietnam War. In addition both periods witnessed a very rapid rise in the divorce rate whereas the years in between showed little change. Divorce rates doubled between 1915 and 1920 and since 1967 the divorce rate has been climbing at about 10% each year. By contrast, the total increase between 1920 and 1967 in the divorce rate was only about 25%.

What is the relevance to the practicing physician of this social science perspective? Basically the relevance is an enhanced sense of understanding the pressures that patients are operating under. At the present time we are at the end of a period of rapid social change in sexuality. Periods of change present increased alternatives to individuals and this often provokes conflict and ambivalence in choices. Patients may come in with psychosomatic symptoms that were precipitated by their struggle with choices regarding sexual behavior or with emotional consequences of sexual behavior they have engaged in. Knowing that this is an exceptional period of rapid change and knowing some of the specific changes going on can help one understand the patients' problems and dilemmas. For example, some married people may feel that they are missing out on mate exchange. Knowing that less than 2% of married couples have tried such mate exchanges (Hunt, 1973) may help in gaining perspective on oneself. One can, of course, go deeper into motivations and potential consequences but this too takes knowledge of (in this case) the sociological studies of "swinging" (Bartell, 1971; Gilmartin and Kusisto, 1973).

CONTRACEPTION AND DOCTORS

The role of contraception in human sexuality is a particularly relevant area for doctors. Modern types of contraception came on the scene about 100 years ago. The event that made the 1876 Philadelphia Centennial famous was not an agricultural exhibit; rather it was the offering for sale at that fair of the first vulcanized rubber condom. Vulcanization allowed for thinner condoms which would not greatly hinder sensation. For decades this device would remain the number one contraceptive method. About the same time (*ca* 1880) the diaphragm was introduced as a contraceptive method. For 80 years these two methods were the best available and even today are used by more people than the pill. They are extremely effective when used properly.

The connection between the advent of modern, highly efficient contraceptive methods and increases in sexual relationships is difficult to establish. First, it should be clear that for all of history most people copulated outside of marriage without benefit of effective contraceptive methods. There always were some known ways of preventing conception ranging from stuffing of rags into the vagina to Casanova's technique of taking one-half of a squeezed lemon and inserting it over the mouth of the uterus (Himes, 1963). The condom itself in animal skin form goes back far before the 19th century. However, only for the past 100 years have highly effective techniques been available and only for a shorter period of time have they been widely known. Even today they are not economically within everyone's ability to purchase. The impact of contraceptive advances on intercourse must then have been quite selective. It is likely that the impact on sexuality for the first few decades after the 1870's would largely be confined to the upper quarter or third of the economic hierarchy, since only such people would be most likely to learn about these methods and be able to afford them. Furthermore, the evidence of the past indicates that the lower social classes were more active sexually before marriage despite their lack of contraception whereas the higher classes were more likely to avoid premarital pregnancy among their own women through the availability of prostitutes. The upper classes were striving to avoid premarital pregnancy in this fashion but there was pressure from the free courtship system that led to opportunity and temptation and thus created a dilemma. The advent of effective contraception helped solve the dilemma by allowing the higher classes to take advantage of the sexual opportunities and yet avoid premarital pregnancy.

Thus, in this limited way, contraception may have encouraged premarital relationships for the higher classes in America. But, for the vast majority, contraception was not a key variable. The prime motivation to sexual intercourse has always been physical pleasure and psychological intimacy. A recent study of a national sample of 15 to 19-year-old girls by Zelnik and Kantner (1972) showed that for the nonvirgins, only between 15 and 20% of these girls *always* used contraception, a similar percentage *never* used it, and the remaining approximately 60% used it only *sometimes*. Clearly, then, much premarital coitus occurs without benefit of contraception and thus contraception can hardly be the key determinant. The knowledge that effective contraception is available may well help encourage sexual behavior and contraception may be used more by older females, but clearly that is only part of the motivational picture.

The 1960's brought two new contraceptive methods—the pill and the intrauterine device (IUD). Here too, the question of how the pill fits into sexual motivation is raised. The evidence on lack of contraceptive use applies to the pill as well. Most of the 15- to 19-year-old females were not on the pill so, clearly, the presence of the pill was not the primary determinant of their sexual behavior. The pill is important primarily because it is a *female controlled* method of contraception. The ancient double standard is still powerful despite the equalitarian gains of the century. Many females not using contraception will say they do not because it is the man's business to contraceptively protect the woman. They hold that the man is the aggressor in sexual relations and should provide contraception (in the form of a condom). The woman pictures herself as submissive and is unable to fully accept the self-image implied by constant use of the pill (constantly available for coitus without the risk of pregnancy). Older women in their 20's are more likely to use the pill, however, and even for younger girls this situation may be changing. But clearly the sexual increases of the late 1960's were not brought on by the presence of the pill. The future may be more affected by it as more and more women come to learn to control their fertility and thereby take a more aggressive sexual stance and decide for themselves what their sex practices will be. Today, we still have many females who play the submissive role and perform sexually because they feel carried away by love or are "seduced" in other ways. The future may well involve more active choice by females.

How does knowledge of contraceptive use relate to the doctor's role with patients? First, it shows that in most cases it will be older and sexually experienced girls that come for the pill. To have gone that far in making a sexual decision is still somewhat unusual for teenage females, although this is probably changing. The doctor can be sensitized to probe for special circumstances when a young female comes for contraception. He can determine to what extent this or any female has thought through her sexuality and to what extent she is playing the traditional female role of doing what her boyfriend wants.

In dealing with public opinion the informed doctor can quickly put to rest fears in the community that the pill is promoting rampant sexuality. In fact, it is well for the doctor to bear in mind that all major studies report that most females are highly discriminant in their choice of a sex partner and that affection and stability of the relationship are still important determinants of the female's sexual behavior. What has happened is that more females have come to accept premarital intercourse when in love, and in a stable relationship (Reiss, 1973). Males visit prostitutes much less than their fathers or grandfathers did and in this sense they too evidence the importance of affectionate ties (Kinsey *et al.*, 1948; Reiss, 1973). However, males still far exceed females in their willingness to accept intercourse as a pleasure which needs no affectionate justification.

Basic human relationships determine sexual occurrences far more than the advent of any contraceptive advance. Such techniques may ease consequences and encourage those on the borderline but they are not fundamental motivators. Knowing this gives the doctor a perspective on sexuality that will encourage open communication with his patients and keep him from accepting mythologies about the relation of contraception and promiscuity.

SOCIAL CLASS AND SEXUALITY

Historical references to social class differences in sexual behavior tend to leave the impression of a lower class that is very high on sexual performance and satisfaction (Gordon, 1973). The image given is that sex is one of the few pleasures available to the poor, and thus they make full use of it. This picture needs serious qualification, at least as it applies to the 1970's.

In the past the lower classes may well have been more sexually active, at least in premarital sex. In part this could have been due to the low sexual activity of the upper social classes, particularly on the part of females. After the advent of modern contraception techniques in the 1870's and 1880's, this situation began to change. As discussed above, it was precisely the upper 25% of the population that was most likely to know of and be able to afford the newer contraceptive techniques. Thus it would be this segment that would in time be encouraged to participate more fully in heterosexual relationships. Females would feel safer once they knew that men had available a method of protecting women from pregnancy. There is still evidence that the lower classes start sexual relationships at younger ages (Rainwater, 1966) but the endorsement of sexuality is more evenly distributed throughout the class system today. The data of Kinsey *et al.* (1948, 1953) gathered in the 1940's showed, particularly for males, greater sexual behavior before marriage by lower class males (on the order of seven times as much premarital intercourse). Nevertheless, the female differences found were heavily related to the age at which sexual relations began. When one compared females who married at the same age and therefore had the same number of years of sexual opportunity, the class differences virtually disappeared. However, black females of the lower social classes were more permissive than upper class blacks (Gebhard, 1958; Reiss, 1967).

In a national sample of adults and a three state sample of high school and college students gathered between March 1959 and June 1963, I probed the relationships between social class and permissiveness in premarital sexuality. There were no significant differences among the social classes in the white group in premarital sexual permissiveness. In the black group there was the older pattern of the lower classes being more sexually permissive. Why didn't I find this traditional pattern in the white samples?

After much testing I found that within each social class there were wide ranges of premarital sexual permissiveness that clustered around the dimension of liberality. By liberality I am referring to the degree to which one favors social change, favors the worth of the individual and favors applying standards equally to all groups. I looked for liberality in the areas of politics, economics, religion, and marriage. If one divided all our respondents into those high on liberality and those low on liberality, striking patterns emerged. Those who were low on liberality displayed the traditional pattern of the lower classes being highest on sexual permissiveness. Those high on liberality displayed a new pattern. Those who were in the higher social classes were the *most* sexually permissive instead of being the *least* permissive. When one put these high and low liberality segments together they cancelled each other out. Thus no relationship appeared between social class and sexual permissiveness in the total samples.

The differences between low and high liberals was particularly sharp in the upper one-third of the social class divisions. My belief is that it was the creation of a high sexual permissive group in the upper one-third of the class hierarchy that has created this new relation of class and permissiveness. This new group in part was a result of the introduction of effective contraceptive techniques and in part a result of other forces. Some of these other forces would be the changes in the occupational system toward jobs that require more self-direction, and more independent judgment (Kohn, 1969). This type of job might well have created a higher likelihood of developing values favoring social change, the importance of the individual, and equal applica- tion of moral rules. The older type of job stressed obedience and conformity and would likely maintain low degrees of liberality. So the new occupational system with its stress on more self-reliant jobs (professional, technical, and managerial jobs have been the fastest growing in this century) may well have promoted liberal values in the upper third of the class system where many holders of these positions are found.

One other point needs to be made here. Rainwater (1966) and other researchers have found that the lower social class has a lower orgasmic rate in their marital sex and reports lower degrees of enjoyment of marital sexuality. This is so although frequency of marital coitus is relatively similar (about three times a week for newly married couples and going down gradually to about once a week by the silver anniversary (Kinsey *et al.*, 1953). Thus, again the image of a hedonistic lower class is not borne out by the research evi- dence. When one notes the abundance of economic hardships and discrimi- nations that the lower classes are burdened with and their known higher divorce rates, it is not surprising to find their sexual lives are not very satisfy- ing.

Now what is the value of this knowledge regarding social class and sexual relationships to the medical doctor? It would be of value to a doctor when a woman presents the symptom of being nonorgasmic in much of her marital sex. If the woman was from the lower classes this lack of orgasm would be more expected for Rainwater's data support such a finding as common. But if the woman is college educated and reports orgasmic failure, then one knows that this is much rarer and more likely reflects causes that are peculiar to that particular marriage or that particular person. The case that fits the social group's sexual pattern can be explained in good measure by group characteristics if one is familiar with the research literature. Thus sociological knowledge is of help in starting the doctor toward an understanding of the patient's individual sexual disturbance. Further, by knowing that social class alone will not afford one sufficient knowledge and that some measure of liberalism is necessary to obtain, the doctor is less likely to misjudge regarding what attitudes of the patient are relevant to an understanding of that patient's sexuality. In short, he should probe attitudes regarding general liberality for they affect sexual attitudes in important ways.

GENERATIONAL DIFFERENCES IN SEX: REAL OR ILLUSORY?

One final area where popular beliefs need to be qualified concerns the question of generational differences in sexual relationships. In my 1963 national sample of 1,500 adults, 21 years of age and older, I compared people of different generations (*e.g.,* 25-year-olds to 50-year-olds). I did find the younger people more acceptant of premarital sexual permissiveness (Reiss, 1967). However, when I then compared people of the *same age* but who were in different roles in relation to marriage, I found much larger differences. In short, the biggest differences were between a 50-year-old male who was single and a 50-year-old male who was married and had a teen-age daughter. Such differences were larger than the differences found when comparing a 50-year-old male and a 25-year-old male. Thus, it seemed that generational change was not as important as was change in one's marital role. When one marries and also when one becomes a parent, and thus responsible for someone else's sexual permissiveness, there is a tendency to become less permissive about premarital sex. The present generation may not demonstrate this lowering of permissiveness as much because it has made its declaration of free choice in sexuality in so outspoken a fashion that it will be difficult to backtrack. But some change, I believe, will occur.

The value of this knowledge to a physician is once more in the area of increasing the doctor's ability to judge the causes of sexual orientations reported by the patient. An unmarried patient may note that although she is 50 years old, she hasn't become any less interested in sexual activity and she may wonder if this is something to be concerned about. The doctor will know that people maintain their acceptance of sexuality and that permissiveness lowers more when it concerns one's child's permissiveness than when it is one's own permissiveness. Such knowledge also helps the doctor to give other patients some insight into changes that may occur after one marries and becomes a parent.

CONCLUSIONS

The basic changes in the last 100 years have been in the direction of more equality between the sexes and a legitimation of the individual's choice of sexual standards. Young people in particular seem to support such a free choice. There appears to have been a constant rise in attitudinal acceptance of these trends although the behavioral increases seem more focused into two periods of time: 1) 1915 to 1920 and 2) 1965 to 1970. The decades between 1920 and 1965 seem to have been decades of consolidation (Reiss, 1960; 1971). The decades that follow the present time may also be a period of consolidation of the behavioral increases that have recently taken place.

There is no physiological barrier to sexual equality. There are cultures in the world where men and women seem equally sexually motivated and thus it must be true that, with specific training, such sexual equality could be achieved. Even in our own country there are vast differences between Mormon youth in college and nonreligious youth in college—clearly such differences cannot be assigned to physiological or hormonal factors but must be accounted for by cultural forces. Knowledge of this sort which indicates that human sexuality has a powerful learned component should make the physician aware that relearning is possible in almost all cases of sexual problems. Rather than perceiving a problem of impotence or frigidity as one fixed by physiology, social and psychological causes will be searched for. While the doctor should of course check for physical causes, the evidence of social science argues that such causes operate in only a small proportion of such cases.

The generally aggressive role of males in most human societies is likely the key determinant of the male aggressive stance in sexuality (Gagnon, 1965). Power and sexuality have a way of going with each other. The group with the greatest political power usually will set up customs that afford it the most sexual pleasures. Physiological differences will take a back seat to such political differences. Here too then, the physician can gain some perspective on his female patients and the causes of their orgasmic patterns.

One other key characteristic of human sexuality in America is the increased tolerance for alternative sexual customs (Reiss, 1971; 1973). This is a key trait of the changes that have occurred during this century and particularly since 1965. This tolerance of life styles fits with the above-mentioned emphasis on freedom of choice and sexual equality. Such a position leads to more openness regarding sexuality and this surely has been characteristic of the last few years in novels, films, and in real life. Perhaps the "living together" customs of the college campuses best indicate this greater openness. This custom is now practiced at one time or another during college by perhaps as many as 25 to 30% of students (Macklin, 1972). A much higher percentage say they accept living together with someone they like or love a great deal and thus this custom is very likely to grow. The physician whose female patient reports living with a male can note the widespread approval by youth of such practices and thereby avoid concluding that he is dealing with an unusual type of person.

Homosexuality, after many years of battling, was taken off the list of categorical psychiatric disorders in 1973. This is in line with cross-cultural evidence (Ford and Beach, 1951) indicating that many cultures in the world take homosexual and bisexual behavior for granted and successfully train their members to act accordingly. Here too the physician is well advised to avoid trying to change his patient's sexual lives into what he thinks is "good" or "normal." It would be more useful instead if a doctor sought for clear signs of physical and mental illness and did not assume such outcomes merely because the patient's sexual life was not in line with the doctor's values. If this can be accomplished in all areas of human sexuality, we will have taken a giant step toward reducing, rather than increasing, the anxiety level in human society.

Social science knowledge can give us awareness of the ranges of human behavior and make us less likely to categorize all behavior of one physical type into one diagnostic category. For example, if one feels strongly that extramarital coitus is bad, then it will be difficult to avoid being judgmental with patients who admit to this. The judgmental physician will also be more likely to diagnose some "abnormality" as the cause or result of this behavior. The sociologist can help control this tendency by pointing out that in the case of extramarital coitus we have marriages ranging all the way from very happy to very unhappy and we have situations ranging all the way from deep love for the next door neighbor's mate to sexual attraction for a prostitute in a foreign country (Christensen, 1962; Cuber and Harroff, 1965; Edwards, 1973). Once we realize the moral complexity of human behavior we will likely hesitate to mix our personal moral judgment with our medical judgment. This clarification of the medical role and the limitation placed on personal moral views are another result that can come from sociological examination. This need not mean that the doctor will endorse as good, any particular sexual act but rather that he will avoid showing condemnation to the patient. A sharper separation of the medical realm and one's private morality is called for. The two realms may mix as when a doctor refuses to perform any abortions because of religious reasons. But it should be clear that this is a private moral choice and not a medical one.

Finally, it should be clear that the trend toward increased sexual permissiveness is not as radical as some would think it to be. To illustrate the scope of the current changes, let me refer to Lars Ullerstam's 1966 book. Ullerstam is a Scandinavian doctor who suggested that we become better "erotic samaritans." To do this he suggested much greater tolerance for the "erotic minorities." He felt that the homosexuals were the most privileged of these minorities and that the child molesters, the voyeurs, and others were much more poorly treated by society. The reactions to this book were critical from many sources. People who would accept the increased amount of adult heterosexual permissiveness were nonetheless nonacceptant of any increased tolerance of these other erotic minorities. Another area is seen in the incest taboo. No one to my knowledge has suggested brother-sister marriage or mother-son marriage. This is considered outside the range of acceptable choices so much that it is hardly even discussed.

All major studies on sexual relationships indicate the very strong emphasis on the value of affection in human sexuality. Most females seem to still endorse this view and more men today than ever before also support the value of affectionate sex (Reiss, 1973). Thus, for most people the trend to more permissiveness has meant an increase in allowable affectionate sexuality.

To be sure, there are some "extreme" advocates such as those who propose mate exchange. But two things must be noted even there. First, "swingers" generally will strongly assert that their first interest is in the preservation of their marital relation and their very entry into swinging is often defended by them as a way of avoiding serious emotional involvements with their extramarital sexual partners. Secondly, I would add that Hunt's recent national survey indicated that less than 2% of the married couples had experienced swinging. Thus, it is hardly a dominant mode of extramarital sexual behavior.

To most people the advantage of the newer attitude to human sexuality is that it affords one a greater opportunity to find a sexual life style suitable to oneself. The older approach to sexuality was more like a Procrustean bed and one was stretched to fit or cut to fit. The major disadvantage of the newer life style is that one may choose unwisely at one point in time and destroy more valuable relationships by seeking momentary pleasures. The stress reactions of the older system would have often been frigidity and the stress reactions of the newer system may well be the inability to control one's sexuality in line with one's major life goals. Groups will differ greatly in these respects. Amish, Mormon, and other highly religious groups may still present the older patterns of problems, whereas many nonsectarian college campuses will more likely present the newer patterns. Every system has its price and it is a private moral judgment as to which system is morally preferable, if any. To achieve discrimination in sex without undue inhibition is what many young people are seeking. They want to discriminate and choose the best sex without feeling inhibited and they want to avoid the lack of goal focus found with indiscriminate sex.

The doctor needs to have some sociological overview if he is to understand the physical and mental problems of his patients. If a patient presents physical ailments related to being overweight, the doctor cannot prescribe treatment unless he first knows how to detect those symptoms and, second, knows enough about the eating habits of Americans to prescribe a new style of eating that is reasonable to follow. The physician also must know the nature of different foods if he is to give the patient a selection of choices that will achieve the same result of solving the overweight problem.

In the case of a patient who presents a sexual disturbance the doctor needs the same things. First, the doctor needs to be able to know when the symptoms are merely the expected ones for the social categories the patient belongs to and when they are quite unusual. He must know the range of behaviors that can be learned and unlearned in order to prescribe. Some overall notion of contemporary trends in sexual relationships affords a perspective on the choices confronting the patient. Only with such sociological understanding can the doctor help the patient see the sexual problem in broad perspective. There are literally millions of Americans with concerns over their sexual life—only if the doctor has an overall grasp of this area of human sexual relationships will he or she be able to reduce anxiety and start the patient on a problem-solving path.

Let us end this chapter on a pragmatic note. I realize that most doctors will not have the time, nor want to take the time, to counsel in depth their patients regarding emotional sexual problems. But even granting that, one can still note that if the doctor has a sound sociological and psychological background in the area of human sexuality, he can make good judgments regarding which cases need to be referred to a specialist. Of equal importance is the fact that with such a background the physician can, by a nonjudgmental and understanding attitude, relieve the anxiety of many patients who need little more than that to go on to solve their own problems.

It would be helpful if medical people would develop a checklist in the area of sexuality that would become part of a complete medical exam. Such a checklist will help take any awkwardness out of dealing with the sexual area. There are short scales developed to measure attitudes toward premarital, marital, and extramarital sexuality that take only a few minutes to administer (Reiss, 1973). I am sure that the doctor who examines a patient's anus has to learn to overcome embarrassment. He is aided in this by such an examination being a routine part of a complete physical and by having key questions that indicate to the doctor whether this is an area in need of further checking. The same is needed in the area of sex.

Of greatest medical importance is the achievement of the goal of reducing sexual anxiety in patients. The 19th century physician succeeded in increasing those anxieties. In the 20th century, physicians will learn more about human sexuality and incorporate sexual histories into medical examinations, and will succeed at reducing anxieties. Most medical people will admit that this is in line with the essential goals of the healing profession. The clarification of these valued goals of medicine and their separation from the physician's private sexual values can be a major impetus to lowered patient anxiety. I believe sociology can make an important contribution here, and it is to that end I dedicate this chapter.

REFERENCES

Bartell, G. 1971. *Group Sex*. New York: Wyden.

Bell, R. and Chaskes, J. B. 1970. Premarital Sexual Experience Among Coeds, 1958-1968. J. Marriage Family 32: 81-84.

Calhoun, A. W. 1945. *A Social History of the American Family*. Vol. 1. New York: Barnes and Noble.

Christensen, H. T. 1962. A Cross-Cultural Comparison of Attitudes Toward Marital Infidelity. Internat. J. Comp. Sociol., 3: 124-137.

Christensen, H. T. and Gregg, C. F. 1970. Changing Sex Norms in America and Scandinavia. J. Marriage Family 32: 616-627.

Comfort, A. 1967. *The Anxiety Makers: Some Curious Preoccupations of the Medical Profession*. London: Thomas Nelson.

Cuber, J. and Harroff, P. 1965. *The Significant Americans: A Study of Sexual Behavior among the Affluent*. New York: Appleton-Century Crofts.

Edwards, J. 1973. Extramarital Involvement: Fact and Theory. *J. Sex Res.* 9: 210-224.

Ehrman, W. 1959. *Premarital Dating Behavior*. New York: Holt, Rinehart and Winston.

Ford, C. S. and Beach, F. S. 1951. *Patterns of Sexual Behavior*. New York: Harper and Row.

Gagnon, J. 1965. Sexuality and Social Learning in the Child. *Psychiatry* 28: 212-228.

Gebhard, P., Pomeroy, W., Martin, C., and Christenson, C. 1958. *Pregnancy, Birth and Abortion*. New York: Harper Bros.

Gilmartin, B. and Kusisto, D. 1973. Some Personal and Social Characteristics of Mate Sharing Swingers. In *Renovating Marriage*. Roger W. Libby and R. Whitehurst, eds. pp. 146-165. Consensus Publications, Dannville, California.

Gordon, M. (ed.). 1973. *The American Family in Social-Historical Perspective*. New York: St. Martin's Press.

Himes, N. E. 1963. *Medical History of Contraception*. New York: Gamut Press.

Hunt, M. 1973. Sexual Behavior in the 1970's. *Playboy* October, pp. 85 ff. Later published as *Sexual Behavior in the 1970's*. Chicago: Playboy Press, 1974.

Kinsey, A. C., Pomeroy, W., Martin, C. 1948. *Sexual Behavior in the Human Male*. Philadelphia: Saunders.

Kinsey, A. C., Pomeroy, W., Martin, C., and Gebhard, P. 1953. *Sexual Behavior in the Human Female*. Philadelphia: Saunders.

Klassen, A., Levitt, E. E. and Reiss, I. L. 1972. Premarital Sexual Relationships. 1963-1970. Unpublished manuscript.

Kohn, M. 1969. *Class and Conformity*. Homewood (Ill.): Dorsey Press.

Krich, A. (ed.) 1963. *The Sexual Revolution: Pioneer Writings on Sex*. New York: Dell Publishing Co.

Macklin, E. 1972. *Cohabitation Research Newsletter*. Department of Human Development, Cornell University, Ithaca, New York.

Malinowski, B. 1929. *The Sexual Life of Savages in Northwestern Melanesia*. New York: Harcourt Brace Jovanovich.

Masters, W. and Johnson, V. 1966. *Human Sexual Response*. Boston: Little, Brown.

Masters, W. and Johnson, V. 1970. *Human Sexual Inadequacy*. Boston: Little, Brown.

O'Neill, W. 1967 *Divorce in the Progressive Era*. New Haven (Conn.): Yale University Press.

Rainwater, L. 1966. Some Aspects of Lower Class Sexual Behavior. *J. Social Issues*, 22(2); 96-108.

Reiss, I. L. 1960. *Premarital Sexual Standards in America*. New York: Free Press.

Reiss, I. L. 1967. *The Social Context of Premarital Sexual Permissiveness*. New York: Holt, Rinehart and Winston.

Reiss, I. L. 1971. *The Family System in America*. New York: Holt, Rinehart and Winston.

Reiss, I. L. 1973. Heterosexual Relationships: Inside and Outside of Marriage. A module for General Learning Press, Morristown, N.J.

Simon, W. and Gagnon, J. 1974. *Research on College Students' Sexuality*. (To be published under a different title.)

Winick, C. and Kinsie, P. M. 1971. *The Lively Commerce*. Chicago: Quadrangle Books.

Zelnik, M. and Kantner, J. F. 1972. Sexuality, Contraception, and Pregnancy among Young Unmarried Females in the U. S. Unpublished manuscript.

chapter

5

Ten percent of the adult male population may be predominantly homosexual. About 5% of adult females may be homosexual (Kinsey et al. 1948, 1953). Many homosexual patients conceal their sexual orientation from physicians due to fear of disapproval and less adequate medical care. Are such fears grounded in fact? Apparently so.

Three-fourths of a sample of a thousand doctors responding anonymously to a questionnaire acknowledged that knowing a male patient to be homosexual would adversely affect their medical management (Pauly and Goldstein, 1970). Clearly, emotional bias, typically myth-activated, contaminates effective medicine.

Much research has been conducted during the past decade comparing and contrasting homosexual and heterosexual life styles. There is considerable overlap between the two. "We are all more human than otherwise." However, unique aspects of a same-sexed orientation also exist. Knowledge of these facts can provide a base from which to understand the homosexually-oriented patient and assure the delivery of our best skills to all our patients.

Editor.

REFERENCES

Kinsey, A. C., Pomeroy, W. and Martin, C. 1948. *Sexual Behavior in the Human Male*. Philadelphia: Saunders.
Kinsey, A. C., Pomeroy, W., Martin, C. and Gebhard, P. 1953. *Sexual Behavior in the Human Female*. Philadelphia: Saunders.
Pauly, I. and Goldstein, S. 1970. Physicians Attitudes in Treating Male Homosexuals. Med. Aspects Human Sexuality 4: 26-45.

The Homosexual as Patient

ALAN P. BELL, Ph.D.

There is no such thing as homosexuality. By this I mean that the homosexual experience is so diverse, the variety of its psychological, social, and sexual correlates so enormous, its originating factors so numerous, that to use the word "homosexuality" or "homosexual" as if it meant more than simply the nature of a person's sexual object choice is misleading and imprecise. When a male or female patient announces his or her homosexuality to the physician, the doctor must conclude nothing more than that the patient becomes erotically aroused by persons of the same sex and/or engages in sexual behaviors with persons of the same sex. As we consider the diversity of homosexual experience, we shall see the crucial mistake in inferring anything more. To put it another way, there are as many different kinds of homosexuals as heterosexuals, and thus it is impossible to predict the nature of any patient's personality, social adjustment, or sexual functioning on the basis of his or her sexual orientation.

MYTHS AND STEREOTYPES

The principal task of the physician, or any helping professional, is to lay aside whatever stereotypes about homosexuals have been picked up along the way and to relate to the patient as an utterly unique human being. It must be remembered that homosexuals, like heterosexuals, are burdened by stereotypes which hardly reflect their status or experience. Many come to believe unfounded assumptions about themselves or to act in stereotypical ways

55

which are not congruent with their deepest needs and feelings. Many remain strangers to themselves and continue to wear masks in the presence of others. Some mouth a rhetoric which is not their own. And it is only in a relationship of trust, in this case marked by the physician's acceptance and appreciation of the patient's individuality, that a human being will come to be surprised by who he is, by what he really wants his life to mean.

Unfortunately, stereotypes of homosexuality die slowly and for a variety of understandable reasons. There are few individuals who cannot recall having heard or read about adult homosexuals who prey upon young boys. Is there anyone who cannot recall a newspaper headline or two which prompted or sustained impressions that homosexuality often involves "dirty old men" in search of innocents, acts of violence, or unimaginable orgies? There may be the memory of a young school acquaintance who did not quite fit into any circle of friends, who could not "cut the mustard" in competitive activities with his peers, and who gave no evidence of any sexual prowess with girls. Such memories can go far in strengthening the association of "homosexuals" with "social misfits."

Perhaps nowhere is the public more tellingly exposed to caricatures of homosexuality than on television, where comedians' jokes suggest that male homosexuals are universally effeminate and female homosexuals (or lesbians) smoke cigars and wish they could play football. In the popular mind, homosexuals of either sex are believed to congregate in certain occupational ghettoes. All male homosexuals are thought to be found dressing hair, decorating interiors, or dancing ballet. Female homosexuals are often portrayed as fiercely competitive and possessed of the most obnoxious aspects of a man's temperament.

In addition to these and other myths about homosexuality to which private citizens in Western countries are exposed, clinicians maintain their own special impressions of homosexuals which can unfavorably affect their relationships with their patients. One common assumption which can be found among helping professionals is that homosexuals are *a priori* "sick." Another is that homosexuals invariably regret their sexual proclivities and would jump at the chance of being "cured." Among the most naive we find the assumption that a shift in sexual orientation is not all that difficult and that all would be different if only the "right person" of the opposite sex came along. Since most professionals come in contact with homosexuals at those times in their lives when they are experiencing psychological or social difficulties, the professionals often feel burdened by the responsibility of doing something about their patient's sexuality. The success or failure of their clinical contacts is then measured on the basis of whether or not a change in orientation has occurred. Such criteria often leave both parties exhausted and dissatisfied with their time together.

There are several reasons, at least, for the distorted views of homosexuality which are held both by the "man-on-the-street" and by those who "should know better." The supposition that there is such a thing as *the* homosexual may stem from a general dislike for complexity of any kind. One's reactions to or attempts to deal with a given group of people are more certain when one can characterize its entire membership in very specific ways. There can be comfort in believing that all blacks or women or married couples or persons living in Appalachia are alike. For many people their self-esteem is momentarily bolstered by characterizing all those belonging to the "out" group in distinctly negative ways. Their need to feel superior to others whose life styles are not like their own makes it well nigh impossible to be objective in their assessments.

In the case of homosexuality, the psychological need of many heterosexuals to view homosexuals with disdain becomes even more understandable. Many persons, uncertain about their own sexual statuses, hang on to the negative myths about homosexuality in an attempt to create distance between themselves and the despised minority. In this way they can at once deny and renounce their own potential for homosexual experience. Who among us does not experience some uncertainty about our sexual selves? Might it not be self-serving to point to a group of people who are sexual failures on more counts than we? Needless to say, what may be excusable among the masses of people cannot be tolerated among those who are preparing themselves for the role of therapeutic agent. The helping professional, committed to the well-being of his homosexual patient or client, must make every effort to become divested of old wives' tales, to replace them with a more realistic imagery, to understand the nature of mental blocks in this area, and to come to terms with whatever psychological needs or conflicts are responsible for a simplistic, chiefly negative, view of homosexuality.

RESEARCH

An important reason for the preponderance of unenlightened views of homosexuality among those in the medical profession is their relative lack of sophistication with respect to behavioral science research. The medical literature is replete with studies of homosexuality employing small, biased samples. Most have been derived from clinical or prison populations and with predictable results: most of the individuals are found to be riddled with psychopathology. The fact that similar results would be obtained with equivalent samples of heterosexuals is suggested by Schofield's investigation (1965). Comparisons between homosexuals and heterosexuals who had been imprisoned, those who had been in therapy, and those who had never sought professional help revealed few differences between homosexuals and heterosexuals in a given category and important differences between those who shared the same sexual orientation but not the same category.

The intelligent reader of research in this area must, at the outset, determine the nature of the homosexual sample. What efforts were made to reach highly inaccessible individuals? How likely is it that the sample will include a diversity of life experiences? In our Institute for Sex Research study (still in progress)—involving both homosexuals and heterosexuals, blacks and whites, males and females—subjects were recruited from several sources: public advertising of various kinds, public and private bars and restaurants where approximately 1,000 hr were spent recruiting potential subjects, small gatherings in people's homes, and contacts made on a one-to-one basis in an effort to reach the most covert individuals. We sent information about the study to almost 6,000 individuals, using the mailing lists of various homophile organizations, bars, and bookstores. We recruited homosexuals in eight steam baths, at the meetings and social activities of 23 homophile organizations, in men's rooms, theater lobbies and balconies, parks and beaches, on the streets, and in public squares. Needless to say, it would have been much easier to rely entirely on the bars or the homophile organizations for subjects, but we wanted to make sure that as many different kinds of homosexuals as possible were included. Without that determination, the incredible range of homosexual experience would have been missing, and we would not have been in a position to delineate homosexual and heterosexual experience more precisely than others have done in the past.

The need to include fairly large samples of homosexuals *and* heterosexuals in studies of homosexuality, to control for a large number of variables in the comparisons which are made, and to understand the nature of "significant differences" between homosexuals and heterosexuals as reported in the literature cannot be stressed too often. Studies of homosexuality which do not include heterosexual control groups are not worth the paper they are printed on. But our concerns should not end here. Whenever comparisons are made between homosexuals and heterosexuals, we must be sure that we are not comparing apples and oranges. They must be equivalent in at least age, education, socioeconomic status, sex, and race. One must employ whatever "statistical controls" are necessary in order to be sure that whatever differences are found cannot be explained by something other than the difference in sexual orientation. For example, a researcher might find that his homosexual sample is more maladjusted—psychologically or socially—than his heterosexual sample, but that when he compares homosexuals and heterosexuals who both report having had a detached father, the difference "washes out." In other words, having a detached father may be far more related to maladjustment then sexual orientation *per se*. Unfortunately, throughout the literature one is apt to find such small samples or such a small number of distinguishing variables that a proper multi-variate statistical analysis cannot be carried out.

Even when the minimal conditions for a valid scientific inquiry have been met, whatever significant differences have been found between a given homosexual and heterosexual sample should not be used by an uninformed readership to construct a stereotype of homosexuality which beclouds important *intra*-group differences. The careful reader of various research reports will often find that significant differences between homosexuals and heterosexuals on a given variable do not even pertain to the majority of the homosexual sample. For example, it might be found in a given study that more homosexuals than heterosexuals did not live continuously with both parents until the age of 17. On the basis of such a finding a reader may conclude that homosexuals are apt to come from broken homes, when in fact most homosexuals in the sample might actually have lived with both parents during the time they were growing up. In the same vein, a higher percentage of homosexuals than heterosexuals may engage in cross-sex dressing. However, it may still be a fact that a distinct minority of homosexuals engages in this activity and, because there are more heterosexuals, that the majority of cross-dressers are heterosexual! One more example: from Bieber *et al.*'s famous study of homosexuality (1962), a great deal has been made of the association between having a detached father and being a male homosexual. The fact is, where Bieber *et al.* found a higher percentage of male homosexuals than male heterosexuals with detached fathers, the majority of both groups had fathers who could be described in this way. In any study one is apt to find a great deal of overlap between the comparison groups, and the careful reader will guard against constructing a stereotype of *the* homosexual (on the basis of statistically significant differences reported between two groups) which does not fit even the majority of the homosexual sample, much less a given individual.

In one's clinical practice it is important that the practitioner keep in mind a number of parameters in the assessment of a patient's homosexuality. During the course of the clinical contact it will become increasingly obvious to the parties involved that any announcement to the effect that "I am homosexual" is not self-explanatory, that such a declaration means different things to and about different people. And only after an exhaustive discussion by the patient of where he or she is with respect to the various dimensions of homosexual experience can a more complete picture emerge. When the assessment includes reference to others' homosexual experience, it can go far in disabusing the patient of his notion that his particular homosexual experience is either inevitable or universal. Hopefully, out of the exchange will come new questions, an awareness of issues which were previously unarticulated, and finally new determinations which are feasible for the individual involved and which reflect a greater understanding of where he is and of where he is going. At the very least, the interest, understanding, and acceptance of an authority figure can go far in helping the homosexual patient recover a fundamental integrity which is sometimes lost coping with the coercive features of a homo-erotophobic culture and the gay world.

THE DEGREE OF HOMOSEXUALITY

One of the first things that must be determined is the extent to which a person's erotic arousal and behavior are homosexual. The matter can be pursued in several ways. In our study we asked respondents to rate themselves on the so-called Kinsey Scale, first with regard to their behaviors and then with regard to their feelings. The scale goes from zero (exclusively heterosexual) to six (exclusively homosexual). It has been estimated that approximately 4 to 5% of American males—and half that percentage of females—are exclusively homosexual (or sixes on the Kinsey Scale) in their behaviors throughout their lives. Additionally, much larger numbers at any given time are exclusively homosexual in their behaviors, and even larger numbers engage in both homosexual and heterosexual acts from time to time. For a given individual, ratings on this homosexual-heterosexual continuum may go up or down depending upon the person's age, life circumstances, and the culture in which he or she lives. It is sometimes helpful to have an individual review his or her behavioral ratings since puberty in order to determine the extent to which he or she has changed over time, the number and nature of the sexual partnerships involved, whatever factors might have accounted for the ebb and flow of homosexual experience, and the various meanings which the individual or others attached to that experience. At what ages was the individual engaging in particular homosexual sexual behaviors? How extensive was the behavioral repertoire? Large numbers of preheterosexual males and females, either before or after reaching puberty, have experiences with members of the same sex which they or others construe as sexual. However, these sporadic experiences usually do not include anal- or oral-genital contact, nor do they involve special emotional feelings for the partner.

The same inquiry should be made with regard to the patient's feelings rating on the Kinsey Scale. Very often the clinician will find that there is not a perfect fit between the two ratings. For example, theoretically it is possible for a person to be exclusively heterosexual in behavior but exclusively homosexual in feeling. Such a person might be married and sexually engaged only with his wife, all the while fantasizing a male partner. The fact that one has less control over one's thoughts and feelings than one's behaviors may be why behavior ratings tend to crowd around the ends of the homosexual-heterosexual continuum, while feelings ratings are spread out more along the scale. Some experts believe that a person's sexual *behavior,* either in the past or at the present time, is a poor indicator of his or her true sexual orientation. They maintain that much more important clues in that regard are provided by a detailed history of a person's sexual *feelings.* Has the individual ever been heterosexually aroused? If so, at what age and how much before or after the first homosexual arousal? Does the person's history include a series of romantic emotional attachments to members of the same sex and explicitly sexual fantasies involving those of the same sex? What proportion of a person's sexual dreams or masturbatory fantasies involve members of the same *vs* the opposite sex? What differences in feelings accompany the individual's homosexual *vs* heterosexual experiences? The majority of homosexual males, and even larger numbers of homosexual females, report extensive heterosexual experience. Many can perform heterosexually, even as adults, but it is a performance frequently bereft of either deep emotional satisfaction or intense sexual arousal.

Out of this inquiry should come an awareness of the extent to which the label "homosexual" is arbitrary. There are females who are multiorgastic with a variety of male sexual partners, but who define themselves as "homosexual" because they find it easier to become emotionally involved with a sexual partner of the same sex. A growing number of females, very much into women's liberation and resentful of their female social status, can be found defining themselves as "homosexual," a definition which amounts to more of a political statement than a "true" indication of their sexual orientation.

Some adolescents think of themselves as "homosexual" because of sexual explorations involving members of the same sex or because they have no particular or exaggerated interest in persons of the opposite sex. Some have been labeled "queer" (*i.e.*, homosexual) on the basis of a lack of interest in sports (if they are male) or an interest in track (if they are female). On the other hand, we know of certain male adolescents who will accept money for blow jobs from older homosexuals but who do not define themselves as "homosexual." There are other males who can be engaged in a variety of homosexual behaviors but who do not define themselves as "homosexual" as long as they do the penile inserting.

Finally, it is interesting to note that in certain cultures there may be found an extraordinary amount of homosexual behavior, but no "homosexuals." The reason for this is that, unlike our own society, homosexuality *vs* heterosexuality is not regarded as an either-or proposition. Adolescents and young adults are not put into the position of having to decide whether they are homosexual or heterosexual. They are free to explore their sexual potential without reference to a rigid classification scheme. Even in our own culture there is a growing number of young persons, sometimes termed "bisexual" or "ambisexual," who refuse to define themselves sexually in highly restrictive ways. They find that they are able to respond sexually, in different ways and on different bases, to a variety of persons, regardless of their sex, and they are unwilling to deny themselves opportunities for sexual exchange out of regard for highly restrictive cultural expectations. In fact, they argue that if it were not for the many repressive features of our society, far more people would become sexually active with persons of both sexes. Many of them believe that their status gives them the "best of both worlds," endowed as they are with capacities for social and sexual intimacy with a great many people whom others are forced to write off as appropriate affectional objects. The bisexual's experience certainly belies the notion that homosexuality and heterosexuality are mutually exclusive. It has challenged a growing number of people—homosexual and heterosexual—to enlarge their capacities for sexual responsiveness. And, of course, in certain circles the person who reports himself or herself to be bisexual is viewed with alarm, often with disbelief. Heterosexuals are apt to conclude that the bisexual is simply on his or her way to an exclusive homosexual orientation, while politicized gays are apt to characterize the bisexual as a "cop-out," giving in to the pressures of a straight society.

In summary, how one defines one's sexual orientation and the basis on which that definition is made differ from one individual to the next, and deserve a great deal of attention before moving into other dimensions of the patient's sexual experience.

LEVEL OF SEXUAL INTEREST

Despite the assumption by the "man-on-the-street" that all homosexuals are constantly preoccupied with sexual thoughts, impulses, and behaviors, the fact is that homosexuals, like heterosexuals, differ in the attention they give to the sexual aspects of their lives. Some eroticize all of their social contacts, and often their sexual engagements become a substitute for genuine intimacy with another human being. Others, probably the majority, go on about their business—of seeking an education or making a living or engaging in various avocational pursuits—with hardly an awareness of their sexual interests. Males, whether they be predominantly homosexual or heterosexual, are more apt to report higher levels of sexual interest than their female counterparts. Homosexuals of either sex who have just "come out," who are in the process of defining their homosexual potential and crystallizing their sexual repertoire, are much more apt to consider sex a very important aspect of their lives or to think about sexual things frequently during the course of the day. As they grow older or more accustomed to the gay scene, these individuals more often than not become less "driven" in their sexual pursuits. A continuing sexual preoccupation can often reflect a lack of suitable sexual outlets or else a dearth of satisfactions from other corners of one's life. On the other hand, the absence of sexual interest may denote a depressive episode, very often triggered off by the disruption of a lover relationship. In the case of the homosexual, categorized on the basis of his or her sexual proclivities, it would not be difficult to understand whatever inclination there is to define the self and others chiefly in sexual terms. And it would be important for the clinician to broaden the homosexual's self-definition as well as the range of his or her interpersonal experience.

SEXUAL STIMULATION

Any appraisal of a person's homosexuality should include a consideration of the kinds of stimuli which are found sexually arousing. The question, "What does he see in her?" which the man asked as he kissed the cow, applies to homosexuals as well as heterosexuals and for as large a number of interesting psychological reasons. More homosexual males than females are apt to report high levels of sexual attraction to persons of the same sex, and it would appear that the less explicitly sexual characteristics of another person (*i.e.,* a good-looking stranger, the bare chest) have a greater stimulus value than those aspects directly associated with sexual activity (*i.e.,* the genitals or buttocks). A composite picture of a sexual partner considered ideal by many male homosexuals would be that of a person who is masculine and youthful in appearance, at least as tall as they are, not overweight, and endowed with a penis of greater than average size. Homosexual females give less emphasis to the physical characteristics which they find desirable in a sexual partner; the few characteristics which they name are apt to include a pleasant face, hair, and eyes, and breasts which are large or of at least adequate size.

It would be important for the clinician to explore the nature of the patient's sexual stimulation, particularly with regard to how restrictive are his or her preferences. The exploration should also include a consideration of the patient's body image as well as whatever remedial steps could be taken to make himself or herself more sexually appealing. At the very least these might include a loss of weight and, among males, a diminution of exaggeratedly effeminate mannerisms.

SEXUAL REPERTOIRE

Again we find that homosexuals can be differentiated with regard to how locked in they are to certain sexual roles and techniques. Some insist on being the penile inserters, others on being the insertees, but clearly this polarization is not characteristic of most homosexuals. Only the most naive researchers or clinicians attempt to classify homosexuals on the basis of such dichotomies as active-passive, inserter-insertee, etc. To be sure, there are preferences, but they are often modified on the basis of the partner's expectations or the individual's sexual interest or arousal. In this country probably the greatest number of homosexual males, after going through a mutual masturbation stage, come to prefer performing fellatio on their partners; a slightly smaller number prefer performing anal intercourse. Among homosexual females one is apt to find a preference for having their sexual partner perform cunnilingus, followed by a preference for being masturbated or for tribadism (body friction which simulates sexual intercourse).

The number of different sexual roles and activities which homosexuals are willing to engage in is often related to their age, to how long they have been involved homosexually with others, and to whether or not they have been involved with other persons who are capable of or interested in sexual experimentation. Frequently, their range of sexual behaviors will reflect the degree to which they accept their sexual impulses and/or homosexual orientation. Sometimes a rigid repertoire will indicate a continuing remoteness from their sexual partners; those homosexuals who risk emotional closeness are more apt to perform sexually in ways that are pleasing to their partners, even if the behaviors do not coincide perfectly with their own special preferences.

The clinician who happens upon a homosexual patient whose sexual repertoire is severely limited would do well to explore the reasons for and consequences of the patient's restrictiveness. It may reflect dominance-submission issues or concerns about being in control of oneself and one's sexual partner or various erotophobic features in the patient which make a wholehearted and spontaneous sexual experience impossible.

LEVEL OF SEXUAL ACTIVITY

In addition to differences in technical preferences, homosexuals differ in the degree to which they are sexually active. Some are satisfied with the frequency of their sexual outlets, while others are not. The latter are apt not to be involved in a relatively permanent sexual partnership and are forced to squander their time and energy in "cruising" (i.e., going out to look for a sexual partner) where successful "scoring" is often not as frequent as many had been led to believe. Some of those who are dissatisfied find it difficult to act in the role of sexual pursuer; they wait to be approached and wooed in a splendid indifference with which they would hide their fears and uncertainty. Some do not know how to cruise, find it difficult to carry out flirtatious conversations, and end up alone in bed or in the bar at closing time. Some wait for a Prince Charming who either fails to appear on the scene or who is whisked off into the night by someone else. Some actually enjoy the "chase" more than the sexual outcome and will sabotage whatever attempts are made to effect sexual closure. The helpful clinician will explore, with his patient, whatever there is about the patient's attitudes or life style that is preventing him from fulfilling his sexual potential.

SEXUAL PROBLEMS

Many homosexuals report that finding a suitable sexual partner is a problem for a variety of reasons: their age, physical attractiveness, their social inhibitions. Some have difficulty maintaining affection for their partners or responding to their partners' sexual requests. Some are concerned with their sexual adequacy: males who have problems maintaining an erection or who cannot ejaculate, females who cannot reach orgasm.

In our society, which does all it can to drive homosexuals underground and to instill fear in those who seek out sexual partners, which endows furtive, impersonal sexual encounters with survival value, and which attempts to inculcate negative views of homosexual behaviors to which homosexuals themselves are frequently not immune, the kinds of sexual problems which many homosexuals report are not at all surprising. Homosexuals for whom their sexual orientation is no longer ego-alien, who have managed to integrate their affectional and sexual needs, and whose sexual partnerships are relatively stable, are apt to report fewer sexual difficulties than those who continue to experience themselves as "odd man out." Regardless, the sensitive clinician should be mindful of these potential difficulties and be prepared to discuss their psychological and social ramifications as well as their possible remedies. He should not conclude that reports of sexual difficulties by homosexuals amount to a general dissatisfaction with their sexual orientation, any more than he would reach such a conclusion on the basis of reports from heterosexuals that they are experiencing sexual problems.

SEXUAL CRUISING AND PARTNERSHIPS

The number and nature of sexual partnerships, as well as the conditions under which they are sought, are important variables within the homosexual experience. Most have experienced at least one "affair" of a relatively long duration, many having lived with the person to whom they were romantically attached and with whom they were erotically involved. For both homosexual males and females such a relationship represents a considerable emotional investment, and its breakdown can have a traumatic effect. For some, and this is more likely to be true of females than males, a permanent relationship of this kind serves as the "be all and end all" of their lives. The first such relationship is sometimes experienced as the first opportunity they have ever had to draw close to another human being, and be accepted for who they are, including their homosexuality. Sometimes one partner will act as a mentor toward the other, introducing him or her to previously unknown features of homosexuality and the gay world. Usually there is the hope that somehow or other the riddle of one's existence will be solved by the relationship, as well as the intention that it will last forever. Sometimes financial resources are pooled, and an entire commitment to the relationship can be reflected in a mutual determination to be sexually monogamous. However, only a small minority ever experience the fulfillment of their original hopes and dreams. More often than not the highly charged sexual atmosphere of the gay world conspires against sexual monogamy. Homosexual males, like their hetero-sexual counterparts, are apt to seek out opportunities for sexual adventure and conquest. In those relationships which preclude sexual freedom for the partners involved, such temptations or activities can provoke a great deal of rancor, guilt, and jealousy. What may be more problematic for the homo-sexual female is an attachment to a person whose sexual orientation is in an unsettled state. It is not uncommon to find an intense female relationship disrupted by a partner who wishes to return to her original heterosexual milieu. Other factors which tend to make homosexual partnerships tenuous are their lack of institutional supports and the fact that a successful relationship makes one's homosexual orientation obvious to family, friends, and em-ployers. In our society long-standing homosexual partnerships can become as much a liability as an asset.

Given such circumstances, the fact that many male homosexuals report having had literally hundreds of sexual partners should come as no surprise, nor should the facts that most of these partners became known to them for the first and last time in connection with one sexual episode, and that most of their sexual encounters involve little care or affection between them and their partners. What must be remembered is that male homosexuals are not provided with the same kinds of institutional supports for their sociosexual liaisons which male heterosexuals enjoy. In the absence of church socials or senior proms or office parties to which the heterosexual male is accustomed, the male homosexual seeks sexual partnerships most often in gay bars, less frequently in steam baths, the streets, private parties, parks, beaches, public toilets, and movie theaters.

A homosexual male's cruising style (an activity hardly worth mentioning in the life of a lesbian) is related to many things. Young homosexuals who have just "come out" or those who have no special partner are apt to cruise more frequently than those who could be categorized differently. Older homosexuals often avoid the bar scene and sometimes rely on the services of male prostitutes if they are not involved in a continuing relationship. Those who are of high economic status and are fearful of being found out will sometimes engage in only the most fleeting sexual encounters in an effort to maintain anonymity. Sometimes such casual and anonymous encounters are a function of a person's inability to relate comfortably to others and a paucity of social contacts. Some who limit their sexual pursuits to a single locale do so because of a long-standing association between sexual arousal and a particular setting. For others it may simply indicate a novice's unfamiliarity with a particular gay community. Again, we find that the homosexual experience can mean quite different things to different people.

Any clinician who would be an influence for good in the life of a homosexual patient would be well advised to become familiar with the social setting of his or her clientele, well versed in the argot of the gay world, and acquainted with a variety of homosexual life styles, some of which are far more productive than others. He should help his patient examine the realism of his expectations *vis-a-vis* a lover relationship and be in a position to help homosexual couples to work through the special difficulties of their relationship. Above all, he should help the homosexual to realize that norms or standards which may be feasible and appropriate for the heterosexual are not necessarily so for the homosexual. Finally, it would be profitable to review the patient's cruising patterns, either in an effort to make them more effective or to reduce the likelihood of harmful social consequences.

OVERTNESS-COVERTNESS

An important area for the clinician to pursue with his homosexual patient is the extent to which he or she is open or secretive about his or her homosexuality. Some homosexuals remain "in the closet," a term used to denote those who lead highly secretive lives. Others reveal their homosexuality only to their closest friends. A growing number of homosexuals are becoming politicized in consciousness-raising groups sponsored by gay liberation organizations and find themselves on picket lines or zapping politicians or certain meetings of the American Psychiatric Association. Needless to say, where one stands on the continuum which extends from the "closet queen" to the gay radical will have a profound effect upon a person's experience of homosexuality.

The most covert individual, sometimes married and often of high socioeconomic status, will frequently limit himself to highly casual sexual encounters in situations where anonymity will be preserved. Such persons will tend to compartmentalize their sexual lives in ways that do them little good. They frequently experience a great deal of tension in pretending to be what they are not, a profound disparity between their inner and outer selves. This fundamental dishonesty leads to a despair that they will never be known to anyone except in a most superficial way. For such people, opening up to a clinician involves a great deal of risk and sometimes marks the beginning of exchanges with others which are more self-revealing than they would otherwise have been. On the other hand, there are homosexuals whose openness is inappropriate and self-defeating, the motivations for which deserve exploration and understanding. Still others feel ashamed that they have not "laid it on the line" and view themselves as moral cowards. Such persons should be led to an understanding that their life situation is unique and that, in fact, on a very deep level their homosexuality is no one else's business. Perhaps only after that becomes their realization will they be in a position to make themselves known to others in ways and on levels which promote their personal growth and sense of well-being.

ATTITUDES TOWARD HOMOSEXUALITY

One's clinical contact with a homosexual is especially important because of the opportunity it provides for the patient to examine his or her attitudes toward homosexuality, either in self or others. The clinician who can communicate a genuine interest, understanding, and acceptance—attitudes which will go far in diminishing the patient's initial defensiveness—is apt to find that the patient has not entirely accepted homosexuality. The possible reasons for such negative attitudes deserve exploration. Sometimes it is because the patient feels that he or she has let down parents, has not lived up to their expectations, and fears their rejection. For some, homosexuality conjures up a host of unacceptable images—"flaming faggots" or "bull dykes," child molesters, lonely adults, or psychological or social misfits—which leads them to false conclusions about themselves and about how life will be for them in the future. Some will have surveyed the literature and come away with the distinct impression that they are outrageously different from the rest of the human race. Sometimes negative attitudes toward homosexuality among homosexuals themselves are the result of social difficulties they have encountered (i.e., arrests, loss of job, blackmail) or of their social isolation even within the gay community. Often negative attitudes will amount to no more than a momentary reaction to the loss of a lover or to a transitory lack of sexual relationships. Frequently such attitudes will reflect more general feelings of worthlessness which have little to do with homosexuality per se.

It is important that the clinician help his patient gain insight into his or her attitudes, first determining whether they are of short or long standing, and then identifying their various sources and the conditions under which such negative attitudes have emerged. The clinician who has no other interest than that of helping the patient to learn where he or she is sexually and knows that certain homosexuals' experiences of their sexual orientation are not inevitable can go far in providing a climate of understanding in which unnecessary burdens can be discarded and from which new attitudes can emerge. This might involve encouraging the patient to read the more recent (and positive) literature on homosexuality (see References) or to participate in a consciousness-raising group sponsored by a gay liberation organization. Usually it will be accompanied by the insight that homosexuality should not be used as the scapegoat for other, even more important, issues in the patient's life which need to be met head on.

PSYCHOLOGICAL AND SOCIAL ADJUSTMENT

For a long time, and for a variety of reasons, many people have supposed that homosexuality is *ipso facto* pathological. The fact is, almost without exception, whenever nonclinical samples of homosexuals are compared with equivalent heterosexual samples, very few, if any, differences are found in their psychological functioning. With regard to their feeling states or self-esteem or various personality characteristics, whether one happens to be predominantly homosexual or heterosexual does not appear to be the crucial variable. Whenever differences are found, they usually do not stand up in other studies, or, as already indicated, the kinds of analyses that are done make it difficult to conclude that the differences are a function of a person's sexual orientation *per se*.

Perhaps more homosexuals than heterosexuals seek professional help or have attempted suicide, but it is as easy to interpret these behaviors as the consequence of being homosexual in a society which is hostile to homosexuality as it is to conclude that homosexuality is caused by psychological maladjustment. From all the evidence we have, one would be hard-pressed not to agree with Hooker's conclusion (1957) that homosexuality—unlike pedophilia or the extreme forms of fetishism, voyeurism, exhibitionism, or sadomasochism—is a sexual variation within the normal range of psychological functioning.

With regard to their social adjustment, again we find occupational, religious, and political differences among homosexuals, as well as differences in the ways they spend their leisure time, the number of friends they have, where they live, and how involved they are in the gay subculture. Very few homosexuals have ever been rolled, robbed, arrested, or fired from their jobs. Much larger numbers report wide circles of friends and a variety of social rewards which they believe to be absent in most "straight" life styles.

CONCLUSION

It has not been my intention to report on the myriad findings about homosexuality which appear elsewhere in the literature. I would encourage the reader to peruse at his or her leisure those works listed at the end of this chapter. What I have tried to do is indicate that homosexuality involves a large number of divergent experiences. These include the *degree* to which one is homosexual, the level of one's sexual *interest* and *activity*, the nature of one's sexual stimulation and *repertoire*, the extent of one's sexual *problems*, the nature of one's sexual cruising and *partnerships*, the degree to which one is *overt,* and the *attitudes* one has toward homosexuality. Homosexuals are found to differ with respect to these dimensions which are themselves related to a homosexual's psychological and social adjustment. Very clearly, there is no such thing as *the* homosexual, and little can be predicted about an individual on the basis of that label.

Only the clinician with this sense of the matter is in a position to help the homosexual client take stock of where he or she is sexually and of where he or she wants or needs to be. Such a clinician will listen carefully to the idiosyncratic statement which the patient is making about self and others by sexual and interpersonal conduct, thereby not only helping the patient to understand the meaning of that peculiar statement, but also leading the patient to an awareness of the panoply of alternative statements and coping behaviors. Regardless of who or where the homosexual happens to be, a clinician who knows what to listen for and really attends to the person sitting across can help that person discover his or her whereabouts. For both people involved, it could come as a surprise.

REFERENCES

Bell, A. P. 1973. Homosexuality, Study Guide No. 2 (revised). Sex Information and Education Council of the United States.

Bieber,, I. *et al.* 1962. *Homosexuality: A Psychoanalytic Study*. New York: Basic Books.

Churchill, W. 1967. *Homosexual Behavior among Males.* New York: Hawthorn Books.

Fisher, P. 1972. *The Gay Mystique: The Myth and Reality of Male Homosexuality.* New York: Stein and Day.

Hoffman, M. 1968. *The Gay World: Male Homosexuality and the Social Creation of Evil.* New York: Basic Books.

Hooker, E. 1957: The Adjustment of the Male Overt Homosexual, *J. Projective Techniques* 21: 18-31. Reprinted in *The Problem of Homosexuality in Modern America.* (H. M. Ruitenbeek, ed.) New York: E. P. Dutton, 1963.

Martin, D. and Lyon, R. 1972. *Lesbian/Woman.* San Francisco: Glide Publications.

National Institute of Mental Health Task Force on Homosexuality. *Final Report of the Task Force on Homosexuality.* Washington, D. C.; U. S. Government Printing Office, 1969.

Saghir, M. T. and Robins, E. 1973. *Male and Female Homosexuality*. Baltimore: Williams & Wilkins.

Schofield, M. G. 1965. *Sociological Aspects of Homosexuality: A Comparative Study of Three Types of Homosexuals*. Boston: Little, Brown.

Weinberg, M. S. and Bell, A. P. (eds). 1972. *Homosexuality: An Annotated Bibliography*. New York: Harper and Row.

Weinberg, M. S. and Williams, C. J. 1974. *Male Homosexuals: Their Problems and Adaptations*. New York: Oxford University Press.

West, D. J. 1968. *Homosexuality*. Chicago: Aldine.

chapter

6

Are there homosexual medical students and physicians? Unless medicine has some special characteristic which repels homosexually oriented applicants, there should be about 20,000 homosexuals in our profession. Do they experience unique problems during training and practice?

Rarely if ever do homosexual physicians reveal themselves to the remainder of the profession. Thus the exceptional nature of what follows.

Editor

The Homosexual
as Physician

HENRY D. MESSER, M.D., F.A.C.S.

The stereotypical idea of the good doctor in our society tends to be the family man who must sacrifice hours that he should spend with his wife and children to take care of the sick or injured patient. Of course, this is often the case. But there are many other types of physicians. Some are female. Some, male or female, love a person of the same sex. Most are equally dedicated and equally concerned.

How many homosexual physicians there may be, no one knows. My guess is that there are about 800 homosexual physicians in New York City alone. This includes female as well as male doctors. Most homosexual physicians are not yet publicly acknowledged and "out of the closet." Only a few are willing to declare themselves and fight for the rights of homosexual physicians within the medical community. Though the medical profession takes a semiofficial attitude that homosexuals are not pariahs, the homosexual physician nevertheless tends to be condemned and looked down on by the great majority of doctors in this country.

Like many homosexual men I know, I seem to have always been that way. I cannot recall any time in my life when I was attracted to the opposite sex more than to the same sex.

I finished at the top of my high school class in a small Southern town and began college at 16. Because I had been so strongly indoctrinated with the "sex is dirty" idea, especially *abnormal* sex, I attempted to completely give up any type of overt sexual activity during college. I believed that it was better to be miserable and do without sex than to be found out and get into trouble. When I got to medical school, I fully believed that I would be thrown out if my true sexual nature were discovered. I am sure that some of my classmates and teachers suspected my homosexuality, but nothing concrete was discussed. I can remember being upset at anti-homosexual remarks and jibes made about three or four faculty members assumed to be homosexual. Yet, some of these same teachers were among the most popular.

Although homosexual teachers appeared to be accepted by some students; other students and young doctors told anti-homosexual stories and jokes. A few doctors even told stories about beating up "queers"—sometimes after leading them on to expect a sexual liaison.

I graduated from medical school when only 22, in 1950, and began interning in New Orleans. Suppressed desires of many years gave way to an easy outlet for homosexual relationships.

Then the Korean War began and I went into the Air Force. The doctor's draft required all young physicians to serve in the medical corps or else be drafted as non-medical soldiers. The enlistment papers required everyone to answer "do you have, or have you every had measles, mumps, scarlet fever, mental disease, homosexual tendencies...etc." Like most homosexual men in those days, I had a terrible dilemma. As Kinsey *et al.* (1948) said "few men with any common sense would admit their homosexual experience to draft boards or to the psychiatrists at induction centers or in the services." The stigma of homosexuality was so great that I denied it on the papers—just as almost everyone else did. Besides, I really wanted to go into the service. I considered it the patriotic thing to do.

Those were the days of Senator Joe McCarthy and the witch-hunts. Homosexuals were called "security-risks" and a great many were discharged from the U. S. State Department. "Communists" and "communist-sympathizers" were weeded out of government service everywhere, and, in the eyes of Senator McCarthy, homosexuals were considered security risks just as were Communists. If they weren't actually subversive, then it was believed they were vulnerable to anyone who found out.

I engaged in an active sex life while in the service, and it was then that I met my lover who has been with me ever since.

While in the Air Force, I was eventually suspected of being homosexual and, after being investigated for 6 months, I was forced to resign my commission and leave the service in disgrace—though no specific act of "wrong-doing" was established. The only factual homosexual contact ever established in the investigation was one that had occurred prior to my entry into service.

As Williams and Weinberg (1971) note, "the manner in which military organizations process their deviant members is a function of the fact that they are able to operate under almost clandestine conditions.... The system is arranged so that the homosexual serviceman is isolated, unprotected, and without the support of others. In the atmosphere created by his exposure he, in effect, discharges himself."

The U. S. military services still pursue strongly homophobic policies. They try to guard the morality of soldiers and sailors by keeping them out of gay bars and away from homosexual contacts. The military establishment seems to prefer that they visit prostitutes or spawn illegitimate babies.

Like nearly every child I had been taught that homosexual activities were wrong—immoral, sinful, dirty, and sick. My straight friends believed it. Naturally, I believed it too. Under those circumstances, one's self-esteem tends to be low.

Before being discharged as a homosexual, I believed that no one really knew about me—unless I wanted them to. After the discharge, it was a public matter. Everyone knew—my parents, friends, and superiors. I had been officially defined as undesirable. One never really gets over that—even when one has learned enough to know that sexuality is basically neither right nor wrong, good nor bad, only variable. One's personal opinion of himself can be made to hit bottom by letting the world convince him that he really *is* sick, or dirty, or sinful, or immoral.

When I was discharged from the Air Force I had already been accepted for a residency in New York City. I came to New York after my discharge from the service intending to explain to the department director what had happened. To my amazement he already knew. I have never found out how. He kept me because he needed my services, but did not recommend that I take the board examinations when I completed my training. When I applied for examination by the board, I was turned down, presumably because of "poor moral character."

Eventually, some of the older men on the board died or retired and were replaced by more progressive-thinking members. I was then allowed to take the examination and passed.

During my days as a hospital resident, I tended to keep my sex life rather secretive, but the fact that I lived with a roommate away from the hospital was not secret. In fact we often gave big parties at our apartment and invited many other house staff members and nurses. These parties were popular and we were well liked. Though there may have been some suspicion of homosexuality, our friends never mentioned it. I believe that when I became chief resident, I was well liked and respected by most members of the house staff, the attending physicians, and the nurses.

I am sure that something of my homosexual background is known to some of the staff and administrators of the three hospitals where I now work. While I have not previously broadcast the story of my sex life, I have made no great attempt to hide it either. I have become progressively more active in the homophile movement, especially the Mattachine Society of New York, and I am convinced that the only way we can dispel the stigma that surrounds us as homosexuals is to make ourselves known as real people who are just as good, capable, kind, concerned, and able as anybody.

Homosexuality *per se* is not illegal (Hoffman, 1968). It is not really against the law to *be* anything. Yet, some 42 states at this time prohibit sexual acts between persons of the same sex. These laws are generally referred to as the "sodomy laws" and they frequently ban a variety of sexual acts between willing participants of opposite sexes—as well as homosexuals. In many states, all oral-genital sexual pleasures are illegal—even between husband and wife.

In actual practice the sodomy laws are virtually never enforced against heterosexual persons. It is only the homosexual who goes to jail for "crimes against nature." Even though one may get away without being caught, the knowledge that one is constantly engaging in illegal sex is demeaning. A climate of fear is ever present. Homosexual men generally believe that the police often go out of their way to be rough on them, a fact which appears to be borne out by objective studies (Niederhoffer, 1967).

For several years I have tried to get the New York County Medical Society to go on record endorsing repeal of the New York State Sodomy law. Such endorsement has already been made by the Association of the Bar of the City of New York, the American Orthopsychiatric Association, the American Civil Liberties Union, the National Association For Mental Health, the American Psychiatric Association, and many other religious and professional groups. Though some committees have reported favorably, the County Medical Society itself has taken no action. If all the "gay" physicians in New York would come out of their closets and knock on the door of the Society demanding action, we would have the votes. But most homosexual physicians are still terrified that their colleagues will consider them somehow unclean, immoral, or even incompetent. A few homosexual physicians have gotten around this stigma by resorting to an essentially all-gay practice—thus withdrawing from heterosexual medicine entirely. This type of practice also reflects the fact that many homosexual patients do not feel comfortable when treated by a heterosexual physician who sometimes may be hostile about the patient's sexual desires.

Although most homosexual physicians lead exemplary professional lives, official medicine has not been in the vanguard of the drive to erase the discrimination and misinformation directed at homosexuality in general, which results in unnecessary suffering. In 1964, the New York Academy of Medicine's public health committee issued a white paper on homosexuality, concluding that it is an illness and may be treated in some instances with improvement and success. No contribution to this white paper was solicited from those who are most intimately knowledgeable about the subject—the homosexuals themselves.

Homosexual physicians must take some responsibility for not writing and speaking on the subject. I admit that I have hesitated to speak out. It takes enormous courage to go before a group of your colleagues and declare that you are what they consider "abnormal," "a dirty old man," "perverted," or at least "sick," and, in the past, most of us have simply lacked sufficient courage. Also, there is the overriding doubt that it would do any real good. It is very easy for one's position to simply be written off because he is a "crackpot" or a "queer." Therefore, of what value is the opinion of a physician who is himself homosexual?

Fortunately, things are gradually changing. Some homosexual physicians are beginning to speak out and some heterosexual doctors are listening. Some organizations are beginning to come aboard. The Psychiatric Society of Westchester County (New York) recently (1973) approved a statement "whereas homosexuality *per se* implies no impairment in judgment, stability, reliability, or general social or vocational capabilities... (we) deplore all public and private discrimination against homosexuals... and urge the repeal of all legislation making criminal offenses of sexual acts performed by consenting adults in private." The Board of Trustees of the American Psychiatric Association, in 1974, voted to remove homosexuality *per se* from the list of mental disorders.

If there are so many gay men and women in medicine, what do they do? What specialties are they in? Do they perform radiology, anesthesiology, and pathology where they would be "safe" from contact with patients? Or do they get into "risky" situations such as pediatrics where they examine little boys and internal medicine where they may take care of men? I know gay doctors in virtually every specialty.

It is no more sexually stimulating for a homosexual urologist to cystoscope a male patient than for a heterosexual gynecologist to use his speculum on a female. Should a homosexual *pediatrician* immediately be suspect? Does one worry about a heterosexual male pediatrician examining infant girls?

I doubt that my private sex life has any effect on my relationship to patients or to patients' families. Except for an occasional homosexual patient referred by a homosexual friend, I do not believe that patients suspect that I might be homosexual. In a surgical specialty like mine, a doctor's private sex life seems irrelevant.

There are also many homosexuals in the nursing profession. They have won a degree of acceptance that doctors have yet to win. No one seems to worry about a gay male nurse bathing a quadriplegic—and indeed, why should one?

Where do homosexual physicians practice? Certainly the big city with its anonymity is sought by many. New York and San Francisco probably have the greatest concentrations. When I leave my hospital in New York City, no one really cares where I go or what I do in the evenings so long as I am available when needed. In a smaller city or rural area, the doctor is expected to show up at the country club or yacht club with his wife, and if he has no wife he simply doesn't fit. Furthermore, if he is suspected of being homosexual he may become an outcast. This is especially true if he prefers not to remain celibate but to pursue the same sexual pleasures available to heterosexuals.

After many years of studying the subject of homosexuality from an intellectual and scientific as well as from a personal aspect, I must conclude that I am an emotionally healthy and stable person, certainly no less so than most heterosexuals. I just prefer a different kind of sexual pleasure than most of the doctors you may know. I think of homosexuality as akin to left-handedness. It is certainly an inconvenience, but not an illness. Drs. Irving Bieber and Charles Socarides would probably tell you that I am sick indeed, that they have seen many mentally ill patients who refused to believe they were ill. By their definition, homosexuality is an illness and that is that. Socarides (1968) states "all homosexuals deeply fear the knowledge that their homosexual behavior constitutes an erotized defense against a threatening masochistic state...." Such an idea is little more than doubletalk. I am not afraid of sex with women. I enjoy it, but it is not my first choice for erotic outlet. I know many homosexual men who are happily married and enjoy sexual relations with their wives—although an occasional homosexual outlet is necessary for complete fulfillment.

How does being homosexual affect a doctor's practice? I must admit, I don't really know. As a surgical specialist, virtually all of my patients are referred to me by other doctors. Probably, there are some doctors who do not refer patients to me because they know or suspect that I am homosexual. However, since I am never even aware of these patients, I have no way of knowing how many there may be—if any. Certainly my practice was set back 10 years by the Specialty Board's refusal to give me their examination. It was almost as though they feared that I might pass and enter their ranks as a known homosexual. When I was finally allowed to take the examination, I was many years out of my residency program and I knew that this entirely verbal examination would be administered by examiners who knew my background. I felt that I had to know the subject matter cold. After receiving my Diplomate, my professional prestige picked up enormously, though my practice has never gotten over 10 years of being boardless. I believe I now have the respect of my colleagues and have become chief of service at one hospital where I work.

Will writing this chapter affect my practice? I certainly hope not, but I suspect it might. Then, why would I accept the Editor's invitation to write it?

As a practicing homosexual, I do not expect to have any biological children. However, I do feel a great responsibility for those who will come after me. I spend a great deal of my time teaching and training young doctors whose sexual orientation is generally unknown to me—but assumed to be predominantly heterosexual. I believe I have a responsibility to help homosexual physicians also. If I can smooth the road for them in any way, it is my duty to do so.

I hope that with this chapter organized medicine will become more understanding. I hope that both homosexual and heterosexual physicians will be made more aware and that the next generation of doctors will treat homosexual men and women more kindly than in the past.

REFERENCES

Bieber, I. and Colleagues, 1962. *Homosexuality, A Psychoanalytical Study.* New York: Basic Books.

Hoffman, M. 1968. *The Gay World, Male Homosexuality and the Social Creation of Evil.* chaps. 5 and 6. New York: Basic Books.

Kinsey, A., Pomeroy, W., and Martin, C. 1948. *Sexual Behavior in the Human Male.* pp. 621-622. Philadelphia: Saunders.

National Institute of Mental Health Task Force on Homosexuality: Final Report and Background Papers. #1724-0244. Available from Superintendent of Documents, U. S. Government Printing Office, Washington, D.C. 20402.

Newsletter, The Psychiatric Society of Westchester, a district branch of the American Psychiatric Association. Section on Psychiatry, Westchester Academy of Medicine, Vol. 15, No. 3, November, 1973.

Niederhoffer, A. 1967. *Behind the Shield—The Police in Urban Society*, Chap. 5. New York: Doubleday & Co.

Socarides, C. 1968. *The Overt Homosexual.* New York: Grune and Stratton.

Williams, C. and Weinberg, M. 1971. *Homosexuals and the Military.* pp. 113-114. New York: Harper & Row.

chapter

7

Christine Jorgensen's "sex change" operation in Denmark, over 20 years ago, generated considerable medical controversy and created a dilemma for American medicine. Some 15 years later, U.S. hospitals began performing similar surgery on persons unable to live in the sex role expected by virtue of their anatomy. However, there is still no agreement on who should be treated with hormones and surgery. More recently, other clinical dilemmas have been created. Dramatic changes have taken place regarding what constitutes appropriately "masculine" and "feminine" behavior.

How are we to counsel patients who want to change sex? What do we tell the parents of a teenage boy who may dress in women's clothes? What advice do we give the parents of a grade-school boy who plays with dolls and wants to be a girl, or the parents of a young girl who refuses to wear a dress and competes with boys in sports?

The area is topical and controversial. Reason has yielded to rhetoric in popular writings and in the placard slogans of social activism. Yet, practical patient guidelines do exist. They are based on empirical clinical facts and accommodate the cultural milieu which envelopes each patient.

Editor

Adults Who Want to Change Sex; Adolescents Who Cross-Dress; and Children Called "Sissy" and "Tomboy"

RICHARD GREEN, M.D.

At an accelerating rate physicians are being confronted by adults who demand to change sex, frightened parents whose adolescent boy has been discovered dressed in women's clothes, and troubled parents of feminine grade-school boys or masculine girls asking whether their child is veering toward homosexuality. What do we know? What can we do?

ADULTS WANTING TO CHANGE SEX

Christine Jorgensen popularized the idea that men who felt like women could "change sex." This was in 1952. For the next decade, as the numbers of men requesting sex change rose, American physicians did little for these people. No centers were evaluating patients or performing surgery. A few physicians (notably Harry Benjamin) were willing to provide estrogenic hormones preparatory to surgery but operations were performed in other countries (primarily Morocco).

In 1965 The Harry Benjamin Foundation in New York initiated a pilot project evaluating preoperative patients. Shortly thereafter, a surgical program was launched at The Johns Hopkins Hospital. When the *New York Times* front-paged the new program, great public and professional interest was generated. At first a few, particularly the University of Minnesota, then several medical centers instituted surgical programs. Thousands of inquiries were received from persons who were casually, moderately, or intensely interested in changing sex.

Nearly all early publicity was for the male-to-female conversion. Christine's surgery, autobiographical accounts such as: *Man into Woman* (1933) (resurrected after the Jorgensen case); *Roberta Cowell's Story* (1955) (an airman from the Battle of Britain becomes an attractive woman), and night club appearances by "sex changes" gave the impression that sex change was an option only for the male. While the latter is not true, the majority of patients requesting sex change have been anatomical males (about 3:1).

Postulated reasons for the unequal number of males requesting sex change are several: 1) the psychodynamic—all children identify first with the most significant other person in their life—mother. Thus the male must disidentify with a female on the road to his male identity, while the female skips that first hurdle toward her femaleness (Greenson, 1967); 2 the sociological—contemporary society affords females more latitude for cross-sexed expression. Females can dress mannishly, live together, and engage in open romantic relationships without the same degree of stigmatization encountered by males. Thus the drive to reduce social alienation by bringing anatomy into conformity with socially accepted patterns of behavior is greater for males; 3) the neuroendocrinological—the basic mammalian state, anatomically, is female and behaviorally may be feminine. Androgen, the masculinizing hormone, is required to produce maleness in the fetus. No sex hormones are required for femaleness (Jost, 1947). Prenatal androgen also appears to influence postnatal behavior in a masculine direction (Young *et al.*, 1964; Ehrhardt *et al.*, 1968). Thus a developmental system (anatomical maleness and behavioral masculinity) requiring the addition of specific amounts of specific substances at critical times is more vulnerable to unfinished or "imperfect" outcomes (*e.g.*, non-masculinized or feminine males); 4) the surgical—construction of a cosmetically acceptable and functional vagina is a more practical goal than is construction of a penis (Jones, 1969; Hoopes, 1969).

More recent popular writings, plus the professional literature, have documented the possibilities of women becoming men. Consequently, more females desperately desiring hormones and surgery are consulting physicians although they remain outnumbered by anatomical males.

General Principles of Management. Key areas of patient management are: 1) evaluating the *motivation* for sex change, 2) evaluating the patient's *understanding* of the *practicalities* of "changing sex," 3) implementing an extended preoperative *trial period*, and 4) for those who undergo surgery, facilitating the period of *postoperative adjustment.*

Persons seek sex change for several reasons, some of which are prognostically good, some poor. Patients may have been misfits as males, not because they are truly feminine but because they are generally misfitted into the greater society. They reason that things can only be better if they harness whatever femininity lies within and live as women. It is unlikely they will do much better in the alternative role. A few other patients are psychotic and delusionally believe themselves to be female, with female internal organs, and perhaps monthly bleeding *per anum* or *urethra*. Acquiescence to such delusional beliefs is risky in that the delusional system may be part of a larger thinking disorder which will remain unaffected or become more diffuse. Additionally, the "transsexual" motive may be related to the degree of the psychotic state at any point in time, with subsequent regret over the genital surgery.

Another patient group is composed of effeminate homosexuals who are victims of the societal discrimination against their behavior and guilt-ridden over being homosexual. They consider that to gain the love they desire from another male, in a social setting which will endorse ṭhat relationship, they must become women. The degree to which these persons have a male homosexual identity rather than a female identity should theoretically weigh against their successfully living as women.

Next, there is the transvestic subgroup. Here, a male, behaviorally masculine during preadolescence, commences cross-dressing with accompanying sexual arousal during teenage, and during adulthood finds cross-dressing and feminine "passing" increasingly comfortable and less erotic. He anticipates a happier future living full time as a woman. On theoretical grounds such persons should be poor candidates for surgery (Stoller, 1968). Their earliest identity was male. The psychodynamic theory of fetishism (sexual arousal to inanimate objects serving as a defense to preserve the penis) also argues against the suitability of such persons for penectomy and castration.* Unanswered questions remain regarding the appropriateness of this group for surgery. To what degree is the waning sexual arousal to cross-dressing a sign that intrapsychic dynamics are changing toward femininity or the general decrement that accompanies most sexual objects (including spouses) with the passage of time? Currently some university medical centers are performing surgery on both these subgroups of patients. Long-term comparative followup with the next type of patient will test the merits of the theory that a transvestic of homosexual history portends poor surgical outcome.

*The reader who wishes to pursue this logic should consult Fenichel's *The Psychoanalytic Theory of Neurosis* (1945). Briefly, the theory holds that the transvestite is unable to accept the existence of penisless people (*e.g.*, mother). He thus creates a "phallic woman" by donning women's clothes. The reassurance that a penis does indeed exist for the woman permits erection.

Finally, there is the group which should have the best prognosis. These are males who from earliest childhood were femininely identified and behaved like girls. Their childhood behavior included cross-dressing, doll-play, role-playing as females, and belonging to a female peer-group. During adolescence and later, they did not find cross-dressing to be sexually arousing. Their sexual attractions from the time of puberty have been directed toward heterosexual males. For these patients whose identity is female, surgery is the finishing touch rather than a sudden leap into femaleness.

What of women who want to become men? Motivations of female-to-male candidates differ somewhat. The occasional psychotic is encountered, as is the behaviorally masculine female homosexual guilty over her erotic fantasies and behavior. However, the female equivalent of the male transvestite is absent. No females report sexual arousal accompanying the wearing of men's clothes.† There are, however, females who felt like boys during childhood and were tomboyish in behavior but, unlike most tomboys, *remained* masculine during teenage. Accompanying the masculinity was a sexual attraction for females. Discriminating these persons from "butch" lesbians (very masculine homosexual females) can be problematic but the critical item is that such lesbians consider themselves masculine females and not men.

Differential Diagnosis. How does the physician determine the motivation for sex change? By asking the patient? Perhaps. That answer is a paradox in medicine. Generally, when we ask a patient about chest pain, shortness of breath, or double vision, we expect accurate, honest answers. But history taking with persons seeking sex change is different. Thanks to the successful promulgation of the professional writings on transsexualism by Benjamin (1966), Stoller (1968), and Pauly (1969), the biographical features of the "true transsexual" are widely known. This literature has been read and thoroughly absorbed more by the transsexual population that the medical. Thus the preoperative patient's expressed purpose in seeking medical help (obtaining sex change) affects the history given. Moreover, it is difficult to obtain cross-validation of these histories by interviewing the person's parents or siblings in that they are typically alienated from the patient or geographically unavailable to the physician.

In consequence of the problems in obtaining an accurate history, clinical emphasis has shifted toward evaluating the patient's present and future, rather than the past. Succinctly put, clinical management says, "If you be-

---

†No fully acceptable answer exists unless one subscribes to the phallic woman theory. In that case, the female is already castrated and has no penis to preserve.

lieve you can function better socially as a female (or male) *prove* it. Dress all day, every day, in the role you desire. Get a job in that role. Move to a new neighborhood and live that new life. See how it really is. You don't need genital surgery now to get a better understanding of what the new life will be." Concurrent with "passing" in the aspired for role, it can be helpful if contrasexed hormones are given. One reaction of the male to high dosages of estrogen will be decreased sex drive and impotence. This should be experienced on a trial basis. Reversible castration (chemical) should precede *ir*reversible (surgical). Breast growth will also begin, a psychologically supporting body change. The knowledge that female hormones are circulating in the blood stream imparts to the patient the feeling that something *is* being done. This trial period permits the patient and physician to gain time, an asset for both (Benjamin, 1966). The trial should last at least a year and preferably two. During this period the male should also undergo the discomforting, costly, and lengthy process of facial hair epilation (electrolysis), a necessary process to facilitate social passing as a woman.

For the female, androgen will lower the voice to a masculine level (the converse vocal change does not occur with males on estrogen). Androgen will also promote the growth of facial hair—a second asset in passing. Additionally, there will be cessation of menses, general body hair growth, and clitoral hypertrophy. The degree of clitoral growth can be considerable, perhaps to 2 inches over a year or so. Another product of androgen administration may be increased sex drive.

One hormone regimen suggested for males is ethinyl estradiol 0.2 to 0.4 mg. a day by mouth with 10 mg. medroxyprogesterone acetate, or estradiol valerate 10 to 40 mg. plus 30 to 60 mg. hydroxyprogesterone caproate by injection, every 2 weeks. For females it can be 250 mg. testosterone enanthate, intramuscularly, every 2 weeks (Benjamin, 1969).

Both male and female patients should understand that they will be infertile after surgery, may not experience sexual pleasure and orgasm (particularly after the male-to-female conversion), and will not be physically indistinguishable from a person who has not undergone genital surgery (particularly after the female-to-male conversion).

Reading materials are available to help the physician, the patient, and the patient's family cope with the problems peculiar to transsexualism. Pamphlet materials are available from the Erickson Educational Foundation, Baton Rouge, Louisiana. More academic material is published in *Transsexualism and Sex Reassignment* (Green and Money, 1969).

ADOLESCENT MALES WHO CROSS-DRESS

No one knows how many teenage males on occasion dress partly or completely in women's clothes with accompanying sexual excitement, never to repeat the behavior during adulthood. Keep this is mind when consulted by the frantic parent and bewildered adolescent. Certainly, most teenagers do not cross-dress, at least not repeatedly, but cross-dressing during that period in life does not mean the person is programmed to lifelong transvestism. A survey of 500 adult transvestites (Prince and Bentler, 1972) found that about half commenced cross-dressing prior to puberty and about half during early teenage. These data do not indicate how many other males cross-dressed earlier in life but abandoned the activity.

The discovery of cross-dressing in a male teenager typically shocks the family in that the boy has heretofore been entirely masculine, with no evidence of "effeminacy." The first bit of clarification which is typically reassuring to the parents and teenager is the statement that cross-dressing does not mean the boy is on his way to a life of homosexuality. Indeed, most transvestites (should this be the outcome) are heterosexual. Second, the relative rarity of adult transvestism weighs against the current behavior as a harbinger of lifelong behavior. Third, transvestism during adulthood is rather effectively treated by behavior modification methods for those who wish to stop. Treatment consists of pairing discomforting faradic stimulation, via a wrist electrode, with fantasies of cross-dressing and actual dressing (Marks and Gelder, 1967).

What causes the adolescent male to wear women's clothes and experience sexual arousal? The etiology is unknown. Perhaps the psychoanalytical theory has some merit, as may Stoller's (1968) description of the mother's unconscious need to feminize her son, or perhaps the learning theorists' proposal of a chance temporal linking of an article of clothing with erotic arousal, an event which is positively reinforced by sexual pleasure, and then repeated (Rachman and Hodgson, 1968).

Phenomenologically, early adolescence for most males is a period of maximal sexual frustration. Genital sex drive is at a new high; available interpersonal outlets are at a low. Masturbation is the primary outlet. Public pornography and private fantasy provide source material to accompany and promote genital arousal. During this period of interpersonal erotic frustration, women's clothes may provide for some males a linkage between the unavailable, interest in the fetish may subside. When a single article of underclothes belonging to a female known to the person (sister or mother) is used for masturbation, the behavior is probably temporary. The cross-dressing drive may be more pervasive for those who dress completely, admire themselves in the mirror, wish others to see them cross-dressed, or resort to stealing women's garments.

How can the cross-dressing behavior be modified when the boy desires change? Should one find that thoughts and practices of cross-dressing are the prime or sole source of erotic excitement, it may be possible to substitute other fantasies. Behavior modification techniques for altering masturbatory fantasies exist. Simply stated, the person begins with the typical, unwanted fantasy and, when sexual arousal is achieved, substitutes a more desirable fantasy and continues masturbation. Over time, the fantasy substitution is introduced earlier during the period of masturbation (Marquis, 1970).

Other management issues focus on "self-destructive" behaviors such as stealing and public exhibiting. The excitement from risk-taking, admixed with self-destructiveness in some patients, hopefully can be interrupted. Sometimes "being caught" is the first public signal by a frightened patient—it is his cry for help.

Inquire also into the boy's fantasies of becoming a woman. Transsexualism can blur with transvestism. The teenage transsexual poses even more of a dilemma than the adult. Many teenage psychiatric "symptoms" are transient and portend little about future behavior. Thus eventual reduction of the transsexual drive is more likely in an adolescent than an adult. In contrast, the onset of puberty and the advent of secondary sex characteristics pose a life crisis. They are dissonant with identity and render him, with each passing month, less capable of subsequent passing as a woman. Male adolescent voice deepening, and facial hair and bone growth propel the would-be-woman further from the biological model of femaleness.

The adolescent transsexual may be behaviorally so atypical for his or her anatomical sex that resultant social ostracism makes daily school attendance an ordeal. The teenager may refuse to continue high school unless permitted to attend in the desired gender role. Realistic, educative discussions with parents concerning the pervasiveness of transsexualism, the need for temporizing procedures for thorough evaluation, and the need for the teenager to *reversibly* test contra-sexed identity can help. These statements can supportively modify their expected incredulity at the thought of their child transferring to a new school, enrolling as a person of the other sex, and (for the male) perhaps having a pubertal slow-down via the administration of estrogen. Some adolescents will do very well in the new role; others will be disillusioned and return. More detailed guidance in this approach is found in Newman (1970).

Additionally, the spectacular cure of one male adolescent transsexual by behavior modification procedures is reported by Barlow *et al.* (1973).

SISSIES AND TOMBOYS

Behavioral Significance. The title of this section hints at the divergent approach to feminine behavior in grade school males and masculine behavior in young girls. "Sissy" is a culturally pejorative term. "Tomboy" is not. Peer group reactions to the two sets of behaviors differ dramatically. Beyond this social significance is a radically different long-range behavioral significance. Consider *first*, that most adult transsexuals recall cross-gender behavior from "as far back" as they can remember, *second*, that three times as many males request sex change, and *third*, that tomboyishness is much more common than sissiness. Thus the probability of a very feminine male continuing with an atypical sexual identity into adulthood is greater than for the masculine girl. Additionally, it is not only the transsexual male who recalls cross-gender behavior during childhood; so did one-half the series of 500 transvestites noted earlier. And, more significant still (because of their greater number in the general population), is the recent report that two-thirds of a series of adult male homosexuals also recalled "girl-like" behavior during childhood (Saghir and Robins, 1973). Finally, there are three follow-up evaluations made during late adolescence or early adulthood of males who had been clinically diagnosed feminine during childhood. Fifteen of 27 were found to be transsexual, transvestic, or homosexual (Zuger, 1966; Lebovitz, 1972; Green and Money, unpublished). Thus, whereas tomboyism is common and in the great majority of cases says little or nothing about later sexuality, very feminine behavior in the young male implies a higher than average probability for later atypical sexuality.

Diagnosis. When is a boy "feminine" to a degree that sexual identity is dramatically atypical? Gender-typed behavior in grade school children is displayed on several parameters: dress, toy preference, activity preference, roles played in fantasy games, peer group preference, and physical mannerisms. The degree of atypical or typical behavior on each parameter must be considered.

We have evaluated over 60 families with atypical boys aged 4 to 10 (Green, 1974). These boys prefer the dress, toys, activities and companionship of girls, role-play as females, display feminine gestures, and may state their wish to be girls. Their cross-dressing began early: in two thirds of the cases, by the fourth birthday, and in all cases by the sixth. It involved genuine or improvised women's attire. A repeated interest in wearing high-heeled shoes has been typically noted, accompanied by the use of jewelry, cosmetics, and other culturally feminine accessories. When genuine articles have not been available, feminine attire has been improvised in a variety of ways: small towels become long hair, large towels become skirts, paper clips strung together become necklaces, crayons and felt-tipped marking pens simulate cosmetics. Cross-dressing is frequent, a typical reply to the question "How often does your son dress up?" is "As often as he can" or "As often as you let him." (Thus, this is not the occasional dressing up of children in nursery school play or on Halloween.) The favorite toy of these boys is a "Barbie" doll or another high fashion doll. They will spend hours with "Barbie," costuming, and recostuming her to the exclusion of all other play. Some parents attempt to divert the boys' interest by substituting "Ken" — "Barbie's" male counterpart. "Ken" is ignored. Rough-and-tumble play and sports, with the exception of swimming, are steadfastly avoided. Girls are strongly preferred as playmates. "Boys play too rough" is the typical cry. When "house," or "mother-father" games are played, the role taken is typically female. "Mother" is the preferred role; if a female playmate insists on being mother, the boy may be "little sister" or "school teacher." Characters imitated from television and films are female: Cinderella, the Wicked Witch, Mary Poppins, and "Batwoman" (not Batman). Gestures may be feminine, including hand and wrist movements when speaking, arm and hip movements while walking or running, and arm, wrist, and shoulder coordination while throwing a ball. Other children call them "sissy." Some boys will say they want to be girls or that they are girls while cross-dressed. "Why?" "Girls get to wear nicer clothes," or "Girls go to nicer places and daddys just go to work" are reasons typically given. Occasionally, there is a more poignant comment such as: "Girls don't have to have a penis."

Thus these boys are atypical on the several parameters of gender-typed behavior for this age group. Their atypical preferences begin during the first years of life and continue on the average for 3 years before consultation is sought. Most parents who bring in their very feminine 7- to 9-year-old boy have been reassured for years by their family doctor: "All boys go through that," "It's just a passing phase," or "He'll outgrow it." While some may, clearly all do not. Discriminating those for whom it is more than a passing phase and signals a heightened probability of atypical adult sexuality is not a simple exercise. It considers each parameter of gender-typed behavior, with respect to *intensity, exclusivity,* and *duration* of cross-gender behavior.

The tomboy is another issue. Most tomboys *will* outgrow it. A few will not. Theoretically, those who will not show cross-gender behavior *and* have a cross-sexed identity. The garden variety tomboy receives some social rewards from the peer group for behaving like a boy; however, she knows she is female (basic sexual identity is female). When social rewards change (with teenage) and positive feedback derives for being feminine, gender-typed behavior changes. It becomes consonant with basic sexual identity. Those few females whose basic identity was not female will respond less, if at all, to changing environmental cues, especially if they discover themselves erotically attracted to females. The above distinction notwithstanding, prospective studies with tomboys are at an embryonal stage and the diagnosis of an enduring tomboy state is hazardous. While occasionally a girl has been evaluated in our study who has given herself a boy's name, has adamantly refused to wear dresses, and has requested surgical construction of a penis (and thus seems more male identified than the usual tomboy), our clinical experience is inadequate to determine the long-term significance of this behavior.

Management. What should the physician do when consulted by parents concerned over their son's "feminine" behavior? First, ascertain the degree to which the boy *is* feminine on the parameters outlined above. Next, consider age. Obviously, the older the boy the more significant the behavior—it has sustained the test of greater time. Similar appearing behavior at age 10 or at age 4 carries different implications. For the parents, the boy's behavior can be put into cultural perspective relative to most boys and girls of that age group. This is frequently helpful for fathers of very feminine boys who may steadfastly refuse to acknowledge that their son is at all atypical. Additionally, parents must not confuse a boy's disinterest in sports and aversion to roughhouse play as being a sign of "abnormality." Further, what is known about the natural course of boyhood feminity can be explained. The little which is known regarding the effectiveness of treatment in promoting change can also be acknowledged. There are no long-term follow-ups of previously feminine boys who underwent psychotherapy during childhood.

Amidst these less than definitive disclosures the child's and parents' current dilemmas can be addressed and help can be given. The boy is usually unhappy. He may want to be a girl and may not comprehend why this is not possible. He may be unhappy over being teased, ostracized, or bullied by classmates. He may be worried that as he gets older he will have no friends because of his behavior. The parents may be receiving criticism from neighbors and teachers because their son acts like a girl. The father may feel he has failed in his responsibility of providing an appropriate male image for his son. The mother may be relentlessly blaming her husband for the boy's behavior: "If you'd only spend more time with him and the family!"

How can we help? Consider first what causes the boy distress. The irreversibility of anatomical sex can be explained with diagrams. The philosophical part of the lesson is that it makes more sense to learn to be happier as you are than to try to be something else. The reasons for peer group teasing can be spotlighted. If they are feminine gestures, avoidance of boy playmates, exclusive doll play, and female role-playing, these can be singly addressed. Boys can be alerted to when they walk, talk, or gesture like girls. For boys in whom this is "automatic," parents can point out to the boy when this occurs. Demonstrations of cultural sex differences in these behaviors can be helpful. If the boy has no male friends because he hates sports and most boys play too rough, male agemates can be found who are themselves not little league enthusiasts or future war heroes. Children may see the world concretely, in black and white. "If I can't do boy things, then I must do girl things." Grays exist: There are boys who do not like rough-house activities, who are esthetic, but nevertheless do not cross-dress, or role-play as female. With some effort by parents, such boys can be imported to provide greater balance in their son's peer group. Gender-neutral board and card games, or handicrafts and art work can substitute for hours with "Barbie" doll. Group male experiences, without an emphasis on sports, can be provided. The gap in the father-son relationship may be closed. Indian Guides, a YMCA program, is a *group father-son* activity with priority given to handicrafts, hiking, and outdoor cooking. Additionally, where parents have been subtly encouraging of feminine behavior, this can be interrupted. The boy may have been receiving positive feedback for cross-dressing or female role-playing in that the behavior is considered cute or funny, and is shown off. Styles of intervention to render these boys happier during childhood and perhaps abort some of the social pitfalls of a continuing atypical sexual identity are reported in *Sexual Identity Conflict in Children and Adults* (Green, 1974).

CONCLUSION

The physician may privately feel that the individual's sexual business is his or her own, providing it does not infringe on the liberties of others.

The physician may also feel that the cultural stereotypes which proscribe and prescribe certain behaviors for males and females are arbitrary and nonsensical. The physician may be appalled at the discrimination which meets persons whose sexual expression is atypical—be they transsexual, transvestic, or homosexual.

While in the public sector the physician may work to attenuate and eventually eliminate these inequities, at the clinical level he must make judgments which are in the patient's immediate best interest. It may seem paradoxical to help an adult male who wants to live as a member of the opposite sex to cross-dress, receive contrasexed hormones, and obtain genital surgery, while on the other hand attempt to reduce extensive feminine behavior in a young boy.

However, the practical goal of clinical management is to reduce social and intrapsychic conflict. At different periods in the life cycle, strategies toward this end differ. Our patients do not live in a vacuum. They and their families are conflicted. As practitioners of a healing art we can help reduce that conflict. This can be approached on two fronts—one clinical; the other political. This chapter outlines a clinical approach to reducing sexual identity conflict in children and adults.

REFERENCES

Barlow, D., Reynolds, E., and Agras, W. 1973. Gender Identity Change in a Transsexual. Arch. Gen. Psychiat. 28: 569-76.

Benjamin, H. 1966. *The Transsexual Phenomenon.* New York: Julian Press.

Benjamin, H. 1969. For the Practicing Physician: Suggestions and Guidelines for the Management of Transsexuals. In *Transsexualism and Sex Reassignment.* (R. Green and J. Money, eds.)

Cowell, R. 1955. *Roberta Cowell's Story.* New York: Lion Library.

Ehrhardt, A., Epstein, R., and Money, J. 1968. Fetal Androgens and Female Gender Identity in the Early-Treated Andrenogenital Syndrome. Johns Hopkins Med. J. 122: 160-167.

Fenichel, O. 1945. *The Psychoanalytic Theory of Neurosis.* New York: W. W. Norton.

Green, R. and Money, J. 1969. (eds.). *Transsexualism and Sex Reassignment.* Baltimore: The Johns Hopkins Press.

Green, R. 1974. *Sexual Identity Conflict in Children and Adults.* New York: Basic Books; London: Gerald Duckworth.

Greenson, R. 1967. Dis-Identifying from Mother: Its Special Importance for the Boy. Paper presented at the International Psycho-Analytic Congress.

Hoopes, J. 1969. Operative Treatment of the Female Transsexual. In *Transsexualism and Sex Reassignment.* (R. Green and J. Money, eds.)

Hoyer, N. (ed.) 1933. *Man into Woman; An Authentic Record of a Change of Sex.* New York: E. P. Dutton, New York: Popular Library, 1953.

Jones, H. 1969. Operative Treatment of the Male Transsexual. In *Transsexualism and Sex Reassignment.* (R. Green and J. Money, eds.)

Jost, A. 1947. Recherches sur la Differentiation Sexuelle de l'embryo de Lapin. Arch. Anat. Microscop. Morphol. Exp. 36: 151-200; 242-270; 271-319.

Lebovitz, P. 1972. Feminine Behavior in Boys. Aspects of Its Outcome. Am. J. Psychiat. 128: 1283-1289.

Marks, I. and Gelder, M. 1967. Transvestism and Fetishism: Clinical and Psychological Changes during Faradic Aversion. Br. J. Psychiat. 113: 711-729.

Marquis, J. 1970. Orgasmic Reconditioning: Changing Sexual Object Choice through Controlling Masturbation Fantasies. J. Behav. Ther. Exp. Psychiat. 1: 263-271.

Newman, L. 1970. Transsexualism in Adolescence. Arch. Gen. Psychiat. 23: 112-121.

Pauly, I. 1969. Adult Manifestations of Male Transsexualism; Adult Manifestations of Female Transsexualism. In *Transsexualism and Sex Reassignment*. (R. Green and J. Money, eds.)

Prince, C. and Bentler, P. 1972. Survey of 504 Cases of Transvestism. Psychol. Rep. 31: 903-917.

Rachman, S. and Hodgson, R. 1968. Experimentally Induced "Sexual Fetishism." Psychol. Rec. 18: 25-27.

Saghir, M. and Robins, E. 1973. *Male and Female Homosexuality*. Baltimore: Williams and Wilkins.

Stoller, R. 1968. *Sex and Gender: On the Development of Masculinity and Femininity*. New York: Science House.

Young, W., Goy, R., and Phoenix, C. 1964. Hormones and Sexual Behavior. Science 143: 212-218.

Zuger, B. 1966. Effeminate Behavior Present in Boys from Early Childhood. J. Pediat. 69: 1098-1107.

chapter

8

"To be or not to be" can reflect on more than suicide. Questions of conception planning, initiation, and continuation clearly predate the later existential dilemma. The physical delivery of population planning devices is covered in standard gynecological and urological texts. Attitudinal delivery is another matter. This chapter is a highly personalized statement directed at a human potential—planning conceptions and births for the purpose of child rearing.

Editor

Conception Control, Birth Control, and Child Rearing

RONALD PION, M.D.

It has been suggested by some that "the population bomb is everybody's baby." Increased attention has been focused in recent years upon the need to include an awareness of "population dynamics" in the medical school curriculum. It is the author's opinion that the subject could and should be treated more relevantly in grades Kindergarten through 12, and by the multimedia comprising the informal system of education. Remedial education, even at a medical school level, will be required as long as sex and reproduction are not considered suitable subjects for earlier study.

Absolute numbers of people on planet earth, counted or estimated at an assigned moment, reflect the relationship between numbers of deaths and numbers of births. The latter figure is derived from the number of coital acts leading to conceptions occurring ± 266 days earlier, minus the number of conceptuses who do not successfully negotiate the intrauterine growth and development phase, for whatever reason.

Neither the "population bomb" nor the majority of conceptions occurring to date was carefully planned. Should the world's people vote for controlled people growth in the future, a variety of belief systems must first undergo evaluation and modification. While this debate develops, it is hoped that medical students might undertake to facilitate conceptions among those anxious to engage in the child-rearing process and facilitate conception avoidance among those not so inclined or committed. Unfortunately, the majority of human conceptions and births occuring during the time it takes to read these thoughts will occur as a consequence of one type of sexual behavior in which humans can participate, namely coitus, or heterosexual intercourse, and not as a result of planning.

The purpose of this presentation is to offer medical students a conceptual framework upon which to build medical practice behaviors that might enable a more relevant response to problems of sexual and reproductive disease. Although each of you has a certain set of points of view, beliefs, and attitudes, all of which are operational within your own value system, nevertheless it is hoped that your mind might be open to a consideration of others.

One belief that has been rather dominant to date ascribes a procreational purpose to the act of coitus. Often accompanying it is the qualifying condition that a couple involved be married prior to pursuing this purpose. To be sure, this dominant theme has been questioned over centuries, but never before in the presence of a communications revolution.

In general, strongly held beliefs change slowly. Groups in power are discomforted and threatened by a process of rapid change, especially when the latter is uncontrolled. The technological hardware for information dissemination has advanced so rapidly in recent decades as to render the continued gradual control of questioned beliefs difficult, if indeed possible.

Strongly held beliefs often require a system of sub-beliefs in order to substantiate the original belief. The rationale for the early evolution of the original belief is often-times lost in translation. Many beliefs have their origins in good ideas which, by agreement and occasionally by confirmation, become accepted.

For example, let us for the moment assume that one of our progenitors observed a need for seeing to it that all infants received proper nurture. This was a good idea. Someone else may have added by observation another good idea, that the nurturing process would be enhanced if the mother devoted much of her time to it. Since she had her own requirements for sustenance, fathers, non-fathers, and non-mothers would then have to provide such sustenance for her. Subsequently rules were developed by those in power to insure the workability of these original good ideas. A reasonable rule may have been established that (biological) fathers should provide the necessary sustenance for mothers who in turn provided the necessary nurturing. Exceptions were of course required when the father was absented by either external cause (death) or internal cause (runaway) and then other men and women, perhaps in the immediate or extended family, would be held responsible for maternal sustenance.

A historical review of many cultural and religious practices supports the reasonableness of the above description and helps the observer to understand the possible origin of rules that govern the sexual and reproductive functions of human beings as they relate to nurturing and rearing practices.

Humans have little difficulty in modifying rules that govern the behavior of domesticated animals, but run head on into great difficulty when attempting to modify a variety of cultural and religious rules that govern their own behavior.

The nuclear family can exert a very positive nurturing influence on the infants born into it, or born out of it but who are reared within it. When families choose to actively participate in the nurturing of infants, results can be and are often positive. It is probable that other carefully designed non-nuclear family systems could also provide the necessary nurturing for the growth and development of human infants. Those interested in designing such systems are free to do so, and are free to evaluate the comparative changes, better or worse, that may be attributable to the experimental design. However, I would like to devote much of my time and effort to the reaffirmation and strengthening of the nuclear family and its potential nurturing power.

It would be well to recognize that faulty nurturing processes probably exert negative influences on the development of children. Child rearing is too important a species function to be carried out by disinterested family members. Competency training might prove helpful but there has been insufficient consensus to date to insure such goal-oriented practices. Hence, children are not always raised by those competent in rearing practices.

THE PROCESS OF CONCEPTION

Conception may be considered artificially as the beginning of child rearing. Conceptions should ideally be undertaken only by those couples desirous of rearing children, but alas, as stated initially, conceptions occur because men and women involve themselves in sexual intercourse.

Sexual intercourse resulting in conception must be accompanied by viable sperm deposited adjacent to the cervix of a woman who has just ovulated or is about to ovulate and produces an egg suitable for fertilization. Some people believe it is at this moment that the "soul" enters the newly created life and further conclude that tampering (inducing an abortion) with this one-celled, binucleated living organism must not be allowed, and that those who tamper (abortionists) are murderers. Some people believe this, I do not.

Not permitting a fertilized ovum to implant is not murder, it is disruption of the implantation site. To the best of our knowledge, all fertilized ova do not implant. To the best of our knowledge, all implanted fertilized ova do not continue to develop. Spontaneous abortion occurs both prior to and after implantation. Intrauterine death may occur and infrequently does anytime during the gestation period. Depending upon its temporal occurrence, it is called spontaneous abortion or miscarriage, intrauterine death, and intrapartum death. Depending upon its temporal occurrence following birth, and depending upon its assigned cause (by agreement), it may be termed a postpartum death, a neonatal death, an infant death, a death, or a murder.

Cattle may be slaughtered, murdered, or their lives terminated. Each word carries a different connotation and, like beauty, is in the mind of the beholder. In some parts of this world, cattle serve as a food source for the human species. Other human beings consider cattle sacred and will not terminate their lives. All life may be considered sacred or not, depending upon one's perspective. The gonococcus is a plant, the redwood is a plant. Some people value the latter, almost no one values the former. People generally arrive at agreement by consensus.

Beliefs persist because of agreement. Conceptions may begin with the full awareness that some 9 months later a child will probably be born. Conceptions may be undertaken exclusively by couples desirous of raising a child. Such a choice is possible by universal agreement.

SEXUAL BEHAVIORS

Sexual excitement and orgasm may or may not be related to conception. Sexual excitement may be considered as but one form of sensual pleasure. Sexual arousal or excitement may or may not be associated with intercourse. Sexual arousal may occur in the absence of another human being. Sexual intercourse may or may not be associated with the deposition of the sperm in the vagina. Assigning a purpose to the act of sexual intercourse is arbitrary. The belief that the act has one major purpose is made by agreement and is also arbitrary.

The feelings and responses associated with sexual arousal may be stimulated in a number of ways. Repetitive association of selected stimuli with a particular response permits conditioning to that response. Those stimuli selected by individuals often are arbitrary. Since learning may be defined as a "relatively" permanent change in behavior, occuring as a result of practice, that which is learned may be modified by practice. That which has not yet been learned may be learned. Each individual is afforded continued opportunities to alter conditioned responses. The process is difficult. However, modification of attitudes and subsequent behaviors is possible.

DEFINITIONS

For centuries, sexual arousal has been associated with recreational and procreational purposes. For centuries, these purposes could be separated or combined.

In Merriam-Webster's Seventh New Collegiate Dictionary, *recreate* ('rek-re-,at) is defined as "to give new life or freshness to," *recreate* (,re-kre-'at) is "to create anew, especially in the imagination"; and *recreation* (,rek-re-'a-sh n) "refreshment of strength and spirits after toil; diversion; a means of refreshment or diversion." *Procreate* ('pro-kre-,at) is defined as "to produce (offspring) by generation, propagate."

Recreation may or may not be associated with procreation, depending upon the intent of the recreational act. Sexual intercourse with deposition of sperm in the vagina is the sexual recreational activity that may lead to procreation. The fact that it need not even when intent *is* specified can be noted in instances of infertility.

Women with congenital absence of the uterus may involve themselves by choice in recreational sexual behavior, including intercourse. They may not be involved procreationally "ever" by choice. They may be involved however in the child-rearing process.

Artificial insemination may be considered as a procreational activity. The sperm donor, whether collecting the specimen during self-stimulation or partner stimulation, can be involved both recreationally and procreationally. Heterologous donors (non-husbands or someone else's husbands) are involved procreationally and recreationally, but are not involved in child-rearing processes. Should the insemination prove successful and procreation begin, an homologous donor (husband) may choose to absent himself from the child-rearing process after birth by divorcing his wife and choosing non-involvement with the offspring.

Refreshing oneself via sexual arousal with or without orgasm can be a responsible individual choice. Ethically, informed consent should be operational when two people engage in sexual recreation. It is preferred that an individual not refresh himself or herself at the expense of the other. Although moral imperatives, by definition, are beliefs, allow me to offer for consideration my belief that individuals *ought not* to refresh themselves sexually or nonsexually at the expense of others.

PREVENTING CONCEPTIONS AND BIRTHS

Pre- and postconception methods that preclude accepting child-rearing responsibilities have been available since the beginning of time (Finch and Green, 1963). As discussed, conception or fertilization requires the immediate proximity of viable sperm and viable egg. Preconceptive methods of fertility avoidance (conception avoidance) require that such a condition (proximity) be avoided. Postconceptive methods of fertility avoidance (birth avoidance) require that the fertilized egg not be transported to the endometrial cavity for implantation. It should not be permitted to implant in the tube or elsewhere in the abdominal cavity in order to avoid ectopic pregnancy. If implanted ectopically, it should be removed to prevent it from damaging the host. Once implanted within the uterine cavity, it can be prevented still from damaging the host either physically or mentally by arresting its development. A number of belief systems attempt to separate mind and body. However, mental damage to a host may be associated with physical damage and physical damage may be associated with mental damage.

Following the birth of a human being, those responsible for nurturing may abandon the child, adopt it out, terminate its life directly or indirectly, or offer inadequate nurturing. Human beings by agreement in varying parts of this world accept different temporal requirements for the duration of the nurturing process. In the United States, the many parents who believe in the importance of continuing education at times will provide nurture, complete or incomplete, through the third decade of life. Empirical evidence exists that some children in the first decade of life, and many in the second, can make it on their own for better and for worse.

ABORTION

Recently, by judicial agreement (Roe *vs* Wade, Supreme Court, January 1973), terminating a pregnancy became a decision to be made by a woman and a physician. Qualifications to this agreement were proscribed and relate to the duration of pregnancy when the act is to be performed.

Multiple points of view are recorded concerning abortion. Some believe it to be murder, others believe it is immoral to compel a woman to continue a pregnancy against her wishes. These two beliefs create a dilemma.

A dilemma may be defined as 1) an argument presenting two or more alternatives equally conclusive against an opponent, 2a) a choice or a situation involving equally unsatisfactory alternatives and 2b) a problem seemingly incapable of satisfactory solution. Thus abortion constitutes a dilemma.

To solve this we can collectively seek innovative methods that might prevent the need for abortion, thus causing the dilemma to disappear. Fail-safe methods of contraception that are preconceptive in design could resolve this dilemma if universally employed. In order for a preconceptive contraceptive method to be fail-safe, it must be responsive to existing attitudes, it must be 100% effective, it must be available, it must be perceived for what it is, and it must be used with responsible choice. No one method developed to date has been perceived or accepted so as to be categorized as totally applicable. For this reason and others, couples and individuals find themselves or their partners pregnant when a pregnancy is neither desirable nor, in some instances, tolerable. When certain points of view are particularly strong, such couples and individuals will utilize rationalization to explain away the problem and accept the undesirable or intolerable condition. Many individuals and couples faced with a similar condition repeatedly have chosen infanticide and abortion even within belief systems that held such acts to be sinful and punishable in either this world or another. A woman desirous of six children may tolerate 10, depending upon her needs and those of the other children, but may draw the line arbitrarily at 11.

A belief system cherishing the value of male offspring may literally force a couple to produce female offspring in order to achieve the highly prized male. Couples, whose earthly possessions are meager and who believe that children are gifts from heaven, may continue to seek such heavenly rewards, even in the face of unmet nurturing needs amongst the children they already have. Males and females who believe it is a sign of their masculinity or femininity to create children may continue to procreate indefinitely. Belief systems that adhere tenaciously to a long-ago pronounced mandate to "be fruitful, multiply, and replenish the earth," (Genesis 1:28) may not recognize the word "replenish" deserves equal weight and consideration, with the *procreative mandate* offered at a time when almost 4 billion people were not here and were not collectively wasteful of this planet's finite resources.

Postconceptive methods that exert their effect after conception are necessary as a back-up to preconceptive method failure, and as a back-up to preconceptive method non-use. Postconceptive methods designed as such might, by agreement, totally replace preconceptive methods. A woman could be allowed to menstruate regularly, whether conception has occurred or not, and especially if the technique could be self-administered, would avoid some problems created by traditional health care systems.

Were awareness of human infant needs more universally proclaimed, associated with a visible commitment to the care of those already here, then people could devote more time to the latter group and philosophize less about facilitating entry from a pre-physical world that may or may not exist.

Another dominant theme present in numerous parts of this world relating to the aforementioned Biblical mandate relates to the presumed need to achieve immortality through procreation. Where is the evidence that immortality is not achievable through rearing a child of other biological parents or through commitment to other human beings? There have been and are individuals who have "put aside" their generational capacity for other pursuits. Those who do this under the cloak of organized religion are considered closer to the divine. Those who do this areligiously often are considered selfish.

STERILIZATION

Permanent methods of contraception, referred to more classically as surgical sterilization, should be available to all individuals who choose not to involve themselves in the child-rearing process, for whatever reason. Such methods should be available, regardless of age, marital status, or any other artificially chosen demographic characteristic, because an individual can make a responsible choice. The responsibility for that choice is the individual's and not that of the health care system, the religious care system, the legal care system, or any other care system.

Rendering an individual permanently nonfertile has most traditionally been carried out by interfering with gamete transport surgically, by removing portions of fallopian tube or vas. Recent research efforts are being directed to altering other parts of the reproductive system and process. For example, ablating the endometrium by some mechanical or chemical method may render a woman both nonfertile and amenorrheic, a condition that some women may find desirable. This latter approach is deserving of a high priority commitment on the part of the scientific community for it could lead to a simple, inexpensive out-patient procedure requiring little in the way of surgical expertise.

PRESENT AND FUTURE CONSIDERATIONS

Some consider the United States today an example of a contracepting society. It is not. Nonprescription contraceptive products are not marketed in the same manner as other nonprescription products. Radio and television commercials advertising condoms, foams, jellies, and creams are essentially nonexistent. The Avon lady does not have such items in her ever increasing "line" of consumer products. They do not appear in the Sears mail order catalogue. The health care system both implicitly and explicitly perpetuates the idea that there are *male* methods and *female* methods and that the pill and the intrauterine device are the most effective methods developed to date. Sex specificity inhibits method adoption. *Couples* should choose, or should not choose, to use methods. Non-coital practices could be substituted at the time of probable ovulation and pregnancy need never occur even in the absence of a responsive or nonresponsive health care system.

It is rather paradoxical that at a time when medical "person power" shortages are being decried and costs of care are rising, family planning activities are being added to a long list of medical responsibilities. Most people interested in avoiding pregnancy as a consequence of sexual intercourse do not need doctors or cumbersome health care systems; they do, however, require information that will provide them with a rational basis for choice and permission to exercise that choice. Rhythm can be used to enhance the efficacy of any couple method, if pregnancy is to be avoided.

Diaphragm fitting rings could be purchased in drug stores or super markets and partners could learn to fit them properly, by carefully studying accompanying pictorial literature. Should any difficulty be experienced during an attempted fitting, the advice that a couple see a physician could be added.

Pregnancy tests could be offered as over-the-counter items to couples anxious to begin a conception or avoid one. This might have the effect of allowing earlier entry to our cumbersome and confusing health care system. False negative and false positive results could be easily explained to the purchaser of the product, again advising medical follow-up for needed clarification.

Our current system of prenatal care, if used, screens for many conditions that could be discovered more profitably prior to pregnancy, rather than in any of the trimesters prior to delivery. Anemias, nutritional disturbances, and other correctable conditions should be treated prior to conception, not afterwards. These suggestions require the commitment of a society to the belief that the human species really is important and that the types of nurturing now offered, systematically and systemically, to certain plants and animals really should be offered to people.

Abortion when necessary should be carried out early. Early means as soon as possible after conception, not at the end of the first trimester. The medical dictionary requires new definitions responsive to consumer needs. The technology exists at present to induce a late menstrual period, hormonally if the woman is not pregnant, and mechanically if she is. Most people in the world do not now know this. The medical community still argues whether the mechanical method should be employed at a time when the diagnosis is uncertain. Interestingly this same group of professionals has for years undertaken surgical means to yield diagnoses, without apology, when the suspected diagnosis has not been confirmed. D and C's have been performed for decades to rule out endometrial cancer or other suspected pathology and when the cancer was not proven, the physician did not apologize for the "unnecessary" procedure. Why should a physician consider apologizing for aspirating a uterus in a woman, sick with anxiety over the possibility of a suspected pregnancy, if he determines as a result of the aspiration procedure that she wasn't pregnant? To be sure hundreds of thousands of consumers should be followed prospectively to ascertain the efficacy, safety and simplicity of the procedure.

In order to have all recognize that menstrual delay among coitally active couples suggests pregnancy, the message must be allowed out of the bag. All preconceptive contraceptive methods at the very least must be accompanied by a product insert suggesting that method failure may occur and if it should, it can be recognized easily by a delay in menses.

Sanitary hygiene products—napkins and tampons—should be accompanied by relevant information describing "how to begin a conception" and "how not to begin a conception, now or ever." Most females universally have their menarche at about age 13 and conceive their first child at about age 17. This descriptive knowledge permits some 4 years to offer pictorial and written information that might substantially alter current reproductive mishaps. A commitment is, however, necessary. The potential for attitudinal alteration is present. Perhaps some decisions will be forthcoming.

REFERENCES

Finch, B. E. and Green, H. 1963. *Contraception Through the Ages.* Springfield (Ill.): Charles C Thomas.

Pion, R. J. 1967. Prescribing Contraception for Teenagers — A Moral Compromise? Obstet. Gynecol. 30: 752.

Pion, R. J. 1969. Pregnancy Detection and Community Outreach, Obstet. Gynecol. 34: 300.

Pion, R. J. 1970. Pregnancy Detection and Community Outreach, in *Population Growth: Crisis and Challenge,* pp. 107-112. Proceedings of the First Population Symposium, University of Wisconsin, Green Bay.

Pion, R. J. 1970. Family Planning: The Family Physician's Responsibility. *Sandoz Panorama,* 8: 18;

Pion, R. J., Wabreck, A. J., and Wilson, W. B. 1971. Innovative Methods in the Prevention of the Need for Abortion. Clin. Obstet. Gynecol. 14: 1313.

Pion, R. J. 1971. Are Abortions Really Necessary? (editorial.) Ann. Intern. Med. 75: 961.

Pion, R. J. 1972. Sexual and Reproductive Planning in Family and Non-Family Units. In *The Family.* Proceedings of the Third Population Symposium, University of Wisconsin, Green Bay.

Pion, R. J. 1972. Preventing Unwanted Pregnancies — The Role of the Hospital. *Postgrad. Med.* 51: 172.

Pion, R. J., Smith, R.G., and Hale, R.W. 1973. The Hawaii Experience. In *The Abortion Experience: Psychological and Medical Impact.* (Osofsky and Osofsky eds.). pp. 177-187, New York: Harper and Row.

chapter

9

Anatomically intersexed infants may be born with genitals so ambiguous that clear visual determination of sex is impossible. In others, genital appearance, while less ambiguous, is contrary to chromosomal configuration, gonadal makeup, or another anatomical determinant of sex. How does one decide whether the infant should be designated male or female? At what age should the decision be made? What should parents be told? Is sexual identity inborn and primarily a consequence of genetic programming, or does it primarily result from postnatal socialization?

Early clinical management precludes the catastrophic personal uncertainty of not knowing whether one is male or female, or feeling that one has been victimized by a trick of nature or a mistake of medicine. This chapter provides guidelines for deciding to which sex the intersexed child should be assigned, when this should be done, and what to tell parents.

Editor

Sex Assignment in Anatomically Intersexed Infants

JOHN MONEY, Ph.D.

CULTURE AND HISTORY

There is an isolated mountain tribe, the Kukukuku, in New Guinea in which a genetic strain of intersexuality has been known to recur (Gajdusek, 1964). Though at birth the affected babies look ambiguous as to sex, rather more feminine than masculine, they are by tradition always assigned as males. The people correctly predict that they will masculinize at puberty, and they are correct, for there is no other strain of intersexuality among them. They predict also that they will need a wife, and so plan accordingly. Again they are correct, for from birth onward they are treated as boys despite their small and defective genitals that require them to sit to urinate.

In our own culture, there are too many different strains or types of hermaphroditism for correct predictions to be made so easily, as in New Guinea, on the basis of inspection of the external genitals alone. The earliest record in our society of how to determine the sex of a hermaphrodite, to use the older and once universal synonym for an intersexed person, is the legal decision of the English jurist, Lord Coke, in the 16th century. He decreed that a hermaphrodite "may be either male or female, and it shall succeed according to the kind of sex which doth prevail." Wisely, he avoided the complexities of trying to define the criteria for ascertaining the prevailing sex. Thereby, he allowed for the person's own decision, a reflection of his own self-knowledge and feeling, to be taken into consideration.

Lord Coke's decision did not provide a guideline for assigning the sex of a newborn hermaphrodite for, in the several strains of hermaphroditism that occur among us, there is no foolproof correlation between external genital appearance and sexualization at puberty. Likewise, there is no foolproof correlation between genital appearance and the differentiation of gender identity, without taking rearing into account.

In the 16th century, the gonads could not be used as the ultimate criterion because they could not always be identified. It was not until the late 19th century, following the discovery of anesthesia and surgical asepsis, that the doctrine of the gonads as the ultimate criterion of sex assignment could be propounded for hermaphrodites. The worship of the tablets of the stones, to make a metaphor from the Elizabethan term for the testicles, became pervasive and, though outmoded, still dictates the decisions of the uneducated and uninformed in hermaphroditism. These same people today sometimes augment or supplant the criterion of the gonads with the criterion of the chromosomes.

On both counts they are wrong, for the correlation between chromosomal sex and gonadal sex with pubertal sexualization and with gender-identity differentiation is as imperfect as it is with genital morphology.

CRITERIA OF SEX OF ASSIGNMENT

Developmental prognosis on the basis of 20th century knowledge of the syndromes of hermaphroditism has replaced the old attempts at prognosis on the basis of classification of hermaphroditic sex according to gonadal or genetic sex. It is now known, for example, that the genetic and ovarian female hermaphrodite with the virilizing adrenogenital syndrome, born with not a clitoris but a penis, will undergo early and masculinizing puberty unless hormonally regulated on cortisone substitution therapy. By contrast, the genetic and gonadal male with the androgen-insensitivity, testicular-feminizing syndrome, born with female external genitalia, is totally incapable of being masculinized even to the most minimal extent, on the basis of today's therapeutics. In hermaphroditic syndromes, the ordinary rules of correlation between genetic, gonadal, and hormonal sex are broken, so that the routine correlations do not hold up, and predictions of somatic and behavioral sexual development cannot be made. To make correct predictions one needs to diagnose the syndrome and know its prognosis.

With respect to psychologic sex and gender-identity differentiation, the criterion of greatest significance in deciding the sex assignment of the intersexual neonate is the criterion of the external genitals. It is quite useless, indeed disastrous, to assign a baby to the sex in which it will never be able to function erotically and coitally, despite the resources of modern surgery and endocrinology.

Pragmatically, this means that an intersexual baby with female-appearing genitals should always be assigned as female. There is no known method of surgery that can reconstruct a clitorine organ into a penile one, nor restore an agenetic or ablated penis. Likewise, there is no hormonal treatment that will induce a hypoplastic organ to enlarge to penile proportions. Moreover, in a significant number of cases of genetic male hermaphroditism in which the phallus is more a clitoris than a penis, failure of the penis to differentiate in fetal life is a manifestation of cellular insensitivity to androgen which will continue to exert its influence at puberty so as to prevent pubertal virilization, allowing the body to feminize instead.

By contrast, a genetically female intersexed baby born with a hypertrophied clitoris may be assigned as a female at birth, even if the hypertrophied clitoris is, in fact, morphologically a penis. In such a case, the external genitalia can be surgically feminized. The internally opening vagina can be exteriorized. Though surgical ablations of the penis leave no clitorine equivalent, erotic feeling and sexual climax are not destroyed. This type of surgical correction must, imperatively, be done neonatally, otherwise, the child will carry traumatic memories of having been castrated; and the parents will not be able to react appropriately to their baby as a daughter, if she has a penis.

In cases of a genetic female born with a penis, there are two options. One is to rear the child as a girl, provided the anomaly is diagnosed and treated very early. The other is to rear the child as a boy, with appropriate removal of internal female organs, eventually, implantation of prosthetic testes, and hormonal regulation of masculinizing puberty. Fetally masculinized genetic females almost invariably develop behaviorally as tomboys, even when reared as girls. Therefore, one can make a strong argument in favor of not neonatally amputating the penis when it has differentiated with a penile urethra in a genetic female. One may instead assign the baby as a boy.

The import of the foregoing discussion of the external genitals is that a child should look like the sex in which he or she is assigned. The child and the parents, to say nothing of relatives and friends, need to be able to see that the genitals do not tell a lie. When there is concordance between genital appearance and sex of assignment and rearing, then in the early years of life gender identity typically differentiates concordantly with both.

MICROPENIS

To achieve concordance between genital appearance, sex of assignment and gender identity is of sufficient moment that, in the case of a genetic male baby born with no penis at all (with the urethra opening in the anus), or with major hypoplasia of the penis, the baby should be assigned as a girl, with appropriate surgical and hormonal intervention. An extremely hypoplastic penis is a micropenis. It may be a skinny tube with a tiny glans and aplasia of the corpora. Otherwise the corpora may be grossly hypoplastic, so that the organ resembles a slightly enlarged clitoris rather than a penis. Technically, it does not qualify as hermaphroditic, because it possesses a penile urethra. But, as in the case of a hermaphroditic, hypospadiac microphallus, it is too small ever to function as a copulatory organ, no matter what surgical and hormonal interventions are attempted.

With or without hermaphroditism, the assignment of a microphallic genetic male baby as a girl does not involve an ethical decision regarding castration and sterility, for the gonads in such cases are typically sterile. Moreover, since they are often undescended, they are subject to enhanced risk of becoming malignant, so that it is advisable to remove them. Left in place, they may or may not masculinize the body at puberty. In some cases the testes feminize, for the body is resistant to their androgen, but not to their estrogen. In these cases, exogenous androgen also has no masculinizing effect. There are some cases also that are associated with growth hormone deficiency and consequent dwarfism of stature which can be partially treated with human pituitary growth hormone. This treatment succeeds, however, in producing an estimated maximum adult height of only 5 ft, more suitable for a girl than a boy.

In borderline cases of microphallus in which the organ appears large enough to function as a small penis, its ability to enlarge and mature at puberty can be tested in infancy. The test consists of applying an ointment containing 0.2% testosterone propionate for 3 months. If the penis shows signs of enlarging, and the pubic hair of growing, then androgen responsivity is established. This procedure is of double value in cases of hypospadiac mircopenis, for it enlarges the organ prior to surgical repair in childhood, and enhances the chances of success. A bigger looking penis also builds the morale of the growing boy and his parents, but with a let-down at puberty. Pubertal enlargement of the penis occurs only once. Thus, if it is induced prematurely by local application of androgen, it does not occur again later when the rest of the body undergoes pubertal development.

ABLATIO PENIS

There are rare cases of traumatic ablatio penis, some as a result of a circumcision accident in infancy. When the penis is totally and completely lost, there is no way of replacing it. Surgically and hormonally, it is possible, however, to rehabilitate the infant as a girl. The first, external repair is done in infancy. The vaginal canal is constructed when the body is fully grown, following pubertal feminization with estrogen, usually around 16 to 18 years. The surgical procedure is similar to that used for genetic females with congenital atresia of the vagina. The ethics of castration in a case of infantile ablatio penis are weighed against the ethics of preserving fertility by exposing a child to live as a boy without a penis, incapable of intromission in adulthood, even if he had the initiative and courage to try a sexual relationship with a partner.

The option of female sex assignment, or reassignment, in a case of ablatio penis is open only in infancy, up to 18 or possibly 24 months of age, by which time gender identity differentiation is already well established. It is impossible for an older child or adult to undergo a voluntary or induced change of gender identity consequent on loss of the penis. The best that can be done, rehabilitatively, in such a case is to prescribe a prosthetic, strap-on penis with which to augment other sexual practices in love making that can be effected without a penis. It is possible to have an orgasm without a penis. The primarey deficit—and destroyer of morale—lies in being unable to satisfy the partner.

THE DAY OF DELIVERY AND AFTER

On the day of delivery, the primary objective in all cases of intersexuality, as in other cases of birth defect, is the rehabilitation of a human life. It is the obligation of all professionals who encounter an intersexual child not to subordinate this objective to their own on-the-spot conjecturing, theoretical vanity, incomplete knowledge, evasive euphemizing, or laissez faire.

Since it is not always possible to decide a newborn hermaphrodite's sex of

EXTERNAL GENITAL DIFFERENTIATION IN THE HUMAN FETUS

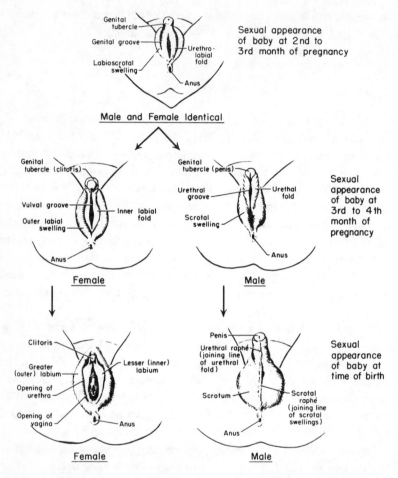

Figure 1. Three stages in the differentiation of the external genital organs. The male and female organs have the same beginnings and are homologous with one another.

assignment by inspection alone, the responsible person in the delivery room is best advised to inform the parents that the baby has unfinished or incompletely differentiated sex organs, and that it will take a few hours, or a few days before the decision can be announced. In this way the parents can play for time before publicly announcing the sex of their new baby and perhaps having later to retract it. Some will decide to confide in their closest relatives; others will decide not to.

SEXUAL DIFFERENTIATION IN THE HUMAN FETUS

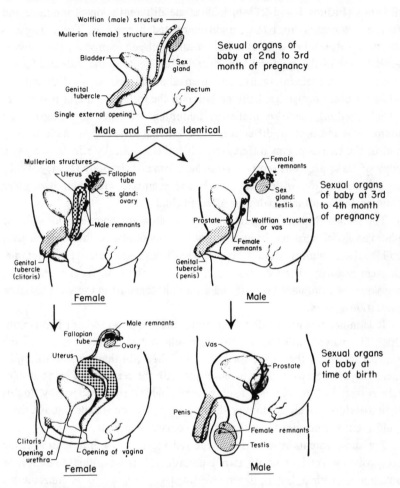

Figure 2. Three stages in the differentiation of the sexual system, internal and external. Note the early parallelism of the mullerian and wolffian ducts, with the ultimate vestigiation of one and the development of the other.

The understanding that parents need most of all concerning their new baby's disability is one that dispels its stigmatization as a freak. Popular stereotypes, which unthinkingly they had grown up with, stigmatize a hermaphrodite (morphodite) as a half-man, half-woman who subsists by being a circus freak. Another popular stereotype, more feared than accepted by the parents, is that their baby's intersexuality is the cause of homosexuality, a condition which they dread and inchoately define.

The first step in destigmatization is best achieved by explanation of the diagrams (Figures 1 and 2) which illustrate differentiation of the male and female sex organs from their undifferentiated beginnings. These diagrams illustrate nature's principle of using the same anlagen to produce the external genital parts of the male and female; and of laying down the male and female anlagen in parallel, internally, and then allowing one set to differentiate, while the other vestigiates. Differentiation of the male set requires that nature adds something, namely, mullerian inhibiting substance to vestigiate the uterus, and androgen to differentiate the internal male organs. With nothing added, the female organs differentiate. It is therapeutically effective to give a copy of these diagrams reproduced in *Sex Errors of the Body* (Money, 1968) to parents for use with their friends and relatives, with their own older children and, eventually, with the affected child.

The second step in destigmatization is to show the parents color slides or photographs of what has been achieved in cases similar to that of their own child. These photos should represent different age levels from infancy through maturity. They should depict details of the genitalia and adolescent physique, and ordinary portrait and group photographs in everyday social or recreational poses.

It is imperative not to dictate by edict the sex of a newborn hermaphrodite. The parents must share the diagnostic and prognostic facts with the experts to whom they look for help. Only then will they be able to implement the decision with full conviction and with the certainty of being absolutely correct in how they are rearing their child. Otherwise, beset by doubt, they are all too likely to convey their anxiety and equivocation about their child's sex, as contagiously as they might convey an infection.

For most parents, the most unexpected piece of new information is the story of how gender-identity is not preordained as masculine, feminine, or ambiguous at birth, but is, like native language, designed to be consolidated under the influence of social exposure and experience. For want of more accurate knowledge, most parents assume, as do most professionals, that little boys are instinctively boyish and little girls instinctively girlish in their behavior, preferences, fantasies, and ambitions. It is an eye-opener to them to learn that, like native language, most of their child's gender behavior will reflect their own expectancy, example, teaching, and reinforcement. Children who underwent fetal androgenization, *in utero,* will, regardless of genetic sex, tend to be tomboyish, behaviorally. Those who underwent de-androgenization will tend to be the opposite. In either case, their tomboyish or untomboyish traits can be incorporated into an overall masculine or feminine gender identity, dependent on sex of assignment and rearing. Their romantic imagery and love affairs in adolescence will, as components of their gender identity, be consonant with assignment and rearing.

Eventually, it will be necessary to counsel parents on the issue of further pregnancies, the sex education of their hermaphroditic child, and how to explain to this child the recurrence of hospital visits and medical examinations. Details vary according to diagnosis, therapy, and prognosis. Before long, the child will be old enough to ask the doctor his or her own questions. For further information, the reader is referred again to *Sex Errors of the Body* (Money 1968). Ideally, one has sufficient time not to have to overload the listener with too much information in one sitting. With children, and sometimes with adults, it is necessary to review information year by year, for the memory distorts and forgets.

SEX REANNOUNCEMENT

It is useful to speak of sex reassignment in older children and adults, and sex reannouncement in the newborn when the change is known to other people, but not the baby itself. The following example of a sex reannouncement is taken from an actual case of a genetic male hermaphrodite with a hypospadiac micropenis. The baby had two aunts with the same condition. They had always been reared as girls, and so successfully that even their brother-in-law, the baby's father, did not know of their condition. Thus he had no precedent to guide him when the obstetrician palpated small testes in the labioscrotum and told the father he had a son. The baby's grandmother recognized the condition as identical with that of her own two daughters at birth. She initiated the referral that ended up in their having to return home in 2 weeks and reannounce the sex, with a change of name from Walter, Jr., to Gwenda.

Several local people already knew that the baby was said to be unable to void. It seemed a good idea, therefore, that the parents continue to tell people that the baby was, indeed, "closed up down there." They would add, however, that when the closed skin was divided, the female organs were revealed, and the baby discovered to be, in fact, a girl. If any explanation was needed about the declaration of the child as a boy, it could be explained that there was an excess of skin on the clitoris.

At the end of their interview on how to deal with sex reannouncement back home, the parents had a good understanding of how and why they had arrived at the decision to have their baby corrected and declared as a girl.

They knew that she could be surgically and hormonally corrected to function as a female in adult life. They knew that she could expect to lead a normal girl's life socially, in romance, marriage, and sexual life with erotic feeling. They knew by contrast, the difficulties, often insurmountable, in trying to correct a baby like theirs as a boy, and the many ways in which the end result might be completely unsatisfactory, even to the point of sexual life being impossible. Above all, they knew at first hand, how successfully the two aunts were growing up, girlishly as girls.

The successful social habilitation of a child after a reannouncement of sex is partly dependent on the way in which the community of which she is a part understands and accepts her. In the isolated and inbred rural area where the parents had been born and near which they now lived, it was necessary to educate the community. The grandmother, who still lived on the farm, and the parents proceeded differently.

The transcription of a taped interview with the grandmother reveals that she had lain awake the night before returning home, trying to think up some way in which to explain the situation to the local people. The opportunity presented itself sooner than she expected. The night of her homecoming proved to be the occasion of the Ladies' Aid Society meeting. She decided to take the bull by the horns and explain the entire set of circumstances to the group of women gathered at the meeting. Asking for the floor after the general business was concluded, she took about 45 min. to explain "the whole thing" to the other women:

"...in plain language like anybody could understand... And they were, oh, they just accepted it and that was it. And I told them, I said, and if you think I've covered up anything you're wrong. I've told you the whole thing, facts. And that was it. I've never had any one of them to approach me any more about it... And I asked them to please explain to their husbands the best they knew how in the words that they could use, no big words, but words that they could use that their husbands could understand. And I haven't had one man to ask me about the child and how it was coming along... I said, I hope I'll never hear any wisecracks made about this child because there's nothing to wisecrack about. I said it's a female. And that's all. And they said, well anybody that would make a crack would be stupid. Since you've explained it to us it's clear. And that was all."

The young parents were relative strangers in the town where they lived. They each decided to give explanations about their baby on a person-to-person basis. They had mentally rehearsed the story so that there would be no mistakes in the telling. The father told most of his fellow employees and close friends.

When asked how many times he had to relate what had happened, he replied with a laugh: "About 200, I would imagine." In spite of the repetitions, he believed it was certainly worth the effort.

The mother felt initially that, even though she had been prepared quite well on what to say, she didn't have the nerve to carry it off successfully:

"...I didn't think I was going to be able to tell it. Until I, well I kept going, you know, the story over and over in my mind. I said well if somebody calls me up I'm not going to be able to tell them. So I called my girl friend—I'm real close with her— and I said well if I can tell her I can tell anybody. So I called her and told her. And after that it just, you know, came easy to me."

Both parents agreed that the situation at home would have been impossible to cope with had they not been fully prepared and briefed on what to do at the hospital beforehand. They believe, as does the grandmother that no further questions have been asked, because they explained the situation exactly as it is. This entire sequence of events augurs well for the baby's future, as the feedback from the community to the child has now been patterned by the explanations given by the parents and grandmother. Should there, in years to come, be any leakage of information about the present crisis, then the parents will not find it difficult to explain in brief and simple terms to the child that, in the presence of an unfinished set of sexual organs at birth, it is very easy to go through a period of uncertainty as to the sex of assignment.

The emotional hurdle of the task confronting this baby's parents and her grandmother is exemplified by the fact that all three of them, despite having been advised to the contrary, omitted any explanation of the baby's sex assignment and name change to the two aunts, Julie and Milly, aged 7 and 5, respectively. Their alibi was that the girls had not questioned them and, therefore, probably had not registered that the baby had originally been declared a boy. Far from it! Both girls were quite articulate in their psychological interviews when the family came to take the baby home. They wanted and needed an explanation, but had correctly recognized the adults' evasiveness and, accordingly, themselves evaded inquiry. The explanation given them was imperative, so that they would know how to behave both now and when their niece would be old enough to talk to them; and also to know that they themselves would be safe from a capricious imposition of sex change.

IDENTIFICATION AND COMPLEMENTATION

The differentiation of gender identity (which in its visible, audible, and feelable aspects is gender role) is jointly the product of identification and complementation. These two processes are reciprocal to one another. In a young boy, to take the example of one sex only, identification takes place when he does or says something, perhaps directly copying his father or other model, that belongs to the stereotype of masculine behavior in the eyes of those who observe it and reinforce it. Those who do the reinforcing may be of either sex. Complementation takes place when this same young boy acts or talks with a girl or a woman in such a way that the pair are taking cues from one another and responding accordingly, each complementing the other in the appropriate sex-stereotypic way. Complementary behavior is also reinforced, and the reinforcing may be by members of either sex.

Complementation takes place, not only with respect to gender roles, but to any roles that are dichotomously stereotyped, for example by age or social status. The special feature of complementation is that, to do it effectively, one must know and anticipate what the other person will say and do in order to know and anticipate what to say and do oneself. With respect to gender-identity differentiation, this means that the masculine and feminine role both become coded in the brain. One is coded positively, so to speak, as a template for personal use. The other is coded negatively, as a template of how members of the other sex behave and need to be reacted to.

A majority of children differentiate their gender identity with fairly clear, non-overlapping boundaries around the schemata of identification and complementation, enclosing within each boundary that which their family and their culture stereotype as masculine or feminine.

The differentiation of gender identity in intersexed children appears to be essentially the same as in other children. One proviso is that intersexed children are more prone to ambivalence, unless the genitals have been made to look appropriate to the assigned sex, perhaps because the parents and others are prone to treat them ambivalently when they appear genitally ambiguous. Another proviso is that genetic females androgenized *in utero* are, as already stated, almost without exception, tomboyish in energy expenditure, dominance assertion, and lack of interest in rehearsing parentalism in play. This type of behavior is, however, widespread among girls in our society and, being an acceptable variant of femininity, is not stigmatizing.

Lack of the boyish counterpart of tomboyism in genetic males deandrogenized *in utero,* though socially more stigmatizing, has not proved a major source of gender-identity disability for boys so affected. These same boys have not manifested a strong degree of parentalism in play. Some have pushed hard to keep up with other boys in competitive sports, finally quitting when they failed to virilize well in adolescence. Despite a very small penis, defective for coitus, some have managed a marriage relationship. There is no doubt, however, that those individuals of the same diagnosis who were lucky enough to have been assigned and reared as girls are confronted with fewer hurdles in making their adjustment to life.

The onset of gender-identity differentiation corresponds with the onset of language development. Language, of course, reflects sex difference in its gender-dimorphic nouns and pronouns. At about 18 to 24 months of age, when a child begins to assimilate these language differences, he begins also to apprehend clothing and other insignia of sex difference. In the third year, he or she, as the case may be, has a clear idea of himself as a boy, or herself as a girl. This is the age at which the core gender identity is said to be established. It becomes so firmly implanted, like native language, that it cannot be eradicated—which is why biological determinists falsely assume that they can attribute all of gender identity to genetics or some other innate inductor.

The strength and tenacity of gender identity, once established, is so great that it will not go away even in the face of a reassignment of sex by edict. The wise rule is: even if the original sex assignment is later deemed a mistake, do not compound the mistake by imposing a sex reassignment after the core gender identity has differentiated. For most children, that means about the age of 18 months. There may be some cases in which a slightly later reassignment can be effected, though not by edict—only after an extensive trial period of preparation in which child and parents rehease the proposed new role.

It is rather rare to find people with a history of corrected intersexuality who are bisexual in either erotic fantasy or erotic practice. Most find themselves heterosexual in their sex of assignment and have no attraction that for them would be homosexual. When bisexualism does occur, it is likely that the intersexual condition was not effectively corrected early in life, or could not be adequately corrected in congruence with the sex of assignment (as used to be routine in cases of the virilizing adrenogenital syndrome in girls prior to the discovery of cortisone therapy in 1950). It is likely also that the parents introduced an element of their own ambivalence and doubt into their child's rearing.

A few intersexed children differentiate an ambiguous gender identity weighted in favor of the sex opposite that of their sex of rearing. Usually it is possible to find a corresponding ambiguity in the rearing, including sometimes an earlier forced reassignment. Typically, the child does not disclose his self-doubt at first, but eventually reaches the decision to change and live as a member of the other sex, on the principle that nothing could be worse than his, or her, present status. The request for sex reassignment is not usually voiced until the child achieves a feeling of teenaged independence. In the earlier years, should such a child be brought to a doctor, he or she may well be too embarrassed and anxiety-ridden to say a word. In counseling sessions, however, the elective mutism may eventually be broken, in writing if not in speaking (Money, 1968).

Requests for sex reassignment in intersexuality have been made by genetic females and genetic males wanting to change from boy to girl and girl to boy, irrespective of genetic sex. In times past, physicians have been inclined to reject requests from genetic female hermaphrodites wanting to live as men, and from genetic males wanting to live as women. Though there are no firm statistics, it may well be that the majority of intersex reassignments in the past have been in genetic males reared as girls. There is probably a sampling bias at work here, for there has in times past been a higher incidence of genetic male babies born and surviving with female-looking genitalia than of genetic females born with male-looking genitals. Genetic male hermaphrodites do not need endocrine therapy with cortisone (available only since 1950) as do most female hermaphrodites, if they are to survive. Further, the parents of genetic male hermaphrodites assigned as girls, through lack of masculine genitals, often have been told about their daughter's testicles in such a way as to feel contradictory confusion about her feminine status, and thus to be ambivalent in their rearing of her.

When a hermaphrodite requests a sex reassignment, the likelihood is that the person has for some time been rehearsing and partly living in the new role, and so is to some extent already rehabilitated in it. Under this circumstance, the transition when the change becomes official is smooth and enduring.

MENTAL HEALTH

The frequency of personality disorder, mild, moderate or severe, in persons with a history of treated intersexuality is probably about the same as in the population at large, though it may be slightly less: the more disturbed the patient's family in its behavioral relationships and the higher the degree of psychopathology in the parents, the greater the likelihood of psychopathology in the intersexed offspring.

A mental health hazard specific to intersexuality in some instances is that entailed in having a body of which the genitals and secondary sexual features do not fit the gender identity. For example, a woman may be excessively virilized, or a man either juvenile or feminized in appearance, and lacking a penis for copulation. Yet, remarkably enough, many individuals so stigmatized have managed to live without the disablement of psychopathology.

Intersexed individuals with a history of effective treatment are habilitated for marriage, and they typically do get married. Female hermaphrodites living as women usually can conceive and carry a pregnancy to term— adrenogenital females only if they are maintained on cortisone therapy. Male hermaphrodites living as males are, in the majority of instances, infertile and so achieve fatherhood either by means of the sperm bank or adoption.

Genetic male intersexes with the complete androgen-insensitivity syndrome have female bodies, live and marry as women and, if they adopt children, become good mothers.

REFERENCES

Gajdusek, C. 1964. Congenital Absence of the Penis in Muniri and Simbari KuKuKuKu People of New Guinea. Abstracts of the American Pediatric Society, 74th Annual Meeting.

Money, J. 1968. *Sex Errors of the Body*. Baltimore: The Johns Hopkins Press.

chapter

10

What is so unique about the female pelvic examination that it requires special focus? Is not this routine examination adequately covered in gynecological texts and amply demonstrated during clinical course work? The contemporary wave of protest by women's groups and the spread of self-help clinics in which women are taught to examine themselves and avoid physicians (of either sex) signals that the situation is short of that desired by many patients.

Many women find the experience of the pelvic examination dehumanizing, degrading, and insensitive. This procedure, vital for the detection of palpable pathology, bacteriological determination of venereal disease, and microscopic screening for malignancy, is an essential component of health care delivery. The pelvic exam must not also be an emotionally alienating experience.

Editor

Pelvic Examination
of Women

DIANE S. FORDNEY SETTLAGE,
M.D., M.S.

This chapter will not describe the multiplicity of pathological findings detected by a pelvic examination. Rather, it will describe those attitudes and techniques of pelvic examination which serve best the patients' need for dignity and the clinician's need for gathering information. It will also highlight those findings which may specifically relate to physical interference with sexual response.

IMPLICATIONS OF THE PELVIC EXAMINATION

Every woman will undergo pelvic examination at some time in her life, and typically a number of times. Very few patients accept the examination calmly, and there are fewer still who do not register more distaste for this exam than for any other routine procedure. Contributing factors are legion, but perhaps the most important are: exposure and manipulation of a person's genitals with the fear of discovery of pathology; violation of body privacy by a person who is at best an awesome, friendly stranger; confusion about the covert and overt sexual overtones of the examination regardless of the sex of the examiner; the expectation of physical discomfort from the procedure; and memories of prior examinations.

For those clinicians who are male, the sensitivity of this exam can best be compared to examination of your own genitals and prostate. Perhaps you have experienced anxiety during penile and testicular manipulation at the time of a physical examination. When the prostate exam occurs, the position is somewhat more humiliating with additional concerns about fecal soiling. The sensation of the rectal exam and prostatic palpation is unusual and uncomfortable, and creates conflict if it is at all similar to sexually related pelvic sensations. Add to your fantasy the same examination by a woman physician, and then evaluate your feelings. Some instructors suggest all male medical students undergo a mock pelvic exam, preferably by a nurse practitioner or woman physician. The students assume the dorsal lithotomy position with legs spread to have the external genitals examined. They are next touched and prodded with a cold speculum along the median raphe, and have a rectal exam and prostatic massage combined with deep abdominal palpation. Such an exercise might help increase sensitivity to the feelings of the woman about to be examined and may help provide a basis for successfully relating to her.

Obviously we cannot explore with each patient the complexities of her feelings (and our own) about the exam. We can, however, alleviate her anxiety and communicate our perception of it verbally: "I understand you are probably a little nervous, at least other patients often are, so let me tell you what I'll be doing."

PREPARATION FOR THE PELVIC EXAMINATION

There are two good ways to prepare for the exam. The preferred is to have the patient disrobed, gowned, covered, and sitting on the examining table when the clinician enters. The medical problem, if one exists, can be explored historically. If the exam is routine, a few minutes can be spent explaining the purpose of the exam. Thus rapport can be established before the patient must lie down on the table and assume the lithotomy position in stirrups. The patient can then be helped to put her feet in the stirrups, while her perineum is covered with a drape. Next, move to the head of the table and help her lie down, holding the drape in position on her abdomen and knee while she moves down to the end of the table with your instruction. Her dignity can thus be maintained by helping her avoid inadvertent exposure during this complicated maneuvering. Concern for her comfort and feelings is established by standing in a location where she knows you are looking at her and not at her genitals. You also do not lose contact with her by leaving the room and then reappearing at the pelvic end of the table. Another good method, but in which the continuity of concern is lost, requires strategic withdrawal while a nurse assists the patient into position.

FACTORS ESSENTIAL TO REDUCING ANXIETY
DURING THE EXAMINATION

The examination begins by palpation of the abdomen. In addition to assessment for abnormalities, this establishes physical contact in a relatively nonthreatening area. Once you have made physical contact, it should not be relinquished until completion of the exam. While changing from the abdominal to the breast exam, let one hand rest lightly on the abdomen as the breast exam begins. Similarly, when beginning the pelvic, contact can be maintained by touching the draped knee and leg. Even if you are not doing a complete physical examination, the second area of exam must include the breasts. Breast cancer is the most common cancer in women, and the breast is emotionally and physiologically a sexual organ which affects body image and body exploration. The breasts are second only to the genitals in provoking examination anxiety. How the patient describes her sensations during that exam, if and when she has discomfort, and her ability to learn breast self-examination provide information about body comfort and sexual anxieties.

Another critical factor in the pelvic examination is the maintenance of eye contact whenever possible. Once the abdominal-leg drape which has been covering the legs and perineum is arranged, having the head of the table elevated about 30° or providing a pillow allows eye contact with the patient while the examiner sits. Depressing the center of the drape, so that it lies flat on the patient's abdomen when her legs are separated, and then folding up the bottom of the remaining drape maintains leg coverage and permits seeing the patient's face.

Throughout the exam, talk to the patient in a natural manner. Inform her of your next task—touching, palpating more deeply, moving to another area, inserting an instrument. Explain what she is liable to feel and tell her to report any discomfort. Encourage her to describe what she feels and to participate actively. A tense patient, for example, will often relax her abdominal and thigh muscles if you encourage her to palpate an area of her abdomen; similarly you can teach and explain the breast exam by having her follow you with her own palpation.

TECHNIQUE OF PELVIC EXAMINATION

Once the abdomino-perineal drape is prepared, move your hand from the knee to the thigh, then to the mons veneris, and finally to the genitals. Inspect and palpate each area of the external genitals while you describe it and your procedure. Elicit concerns or complaints about each area as you proceed. In examining the patient with a sexual dysfunction, observe carefully for evidence of mucous membrane color change, physiological engorgement of the clitoris and labia minora, and quantitative change in vaginal secretions as you proceed. These parameters of early sexual response can and do occur during the course of a thorough exam in many patients. They are invaluable in establishing the presence of an intact afferent and efferent neurological reflex arc.

External Genitals

The clitoris should be palpated for assessment of its anatomical diameters and their normalcy. The clitoral prepuce should be retracted and its juncture with the clitoris examined for signs of inflammation, smegma, lesions, and adhesions. Some authors (Hartman and Fithian, 1973) report a high incidence of clitoral adhesions in anorgasmic women. My own experience supports the rare finding of adhesions with no ascertainable relationship to anorgasmic etiology, and invariable occurrence of clitoral complaints when adhesions are found. It is much more common to find evidence of smegma or minor inflammation which may contribute to a sexual problem but is not etiological.

Similarly, the labia minora should be palpated and inspected for lesions, varicosities, and inflammation which may be localized or diffuse. Women may have concerns about inequality of size or shape of a labium minus which reflect neither anatomical pathology nor dysfunction etiology but do reflect on body imagery and masturbation anxiety.

Examination of the perineal body and introitus of the vagina can reveal conditions which contribute to inadequate sexual function. Small fissures, abrasions, and erythema may indicate chronic vulvitis contributing to, or resultant of, dyspareunia (painful intercourse) and sexual avoidance. Old scars or palpably firm areas associated with pain on examination may relate to similar problems. A perineal body which is very narrow, so that the vaginal introitus is gaping, may indicate lack of sensation and anorgasmia (or partner complaints) because of inadequate function of the pubococcygeus muscle. Insertion of two fingers into the distal vagina and palpation of the muscles forming the levator sling will identify atrophy or midline separation of these muscles. Asking the patient to squeeze your fingers helps to evaluate muscle tone, muscle defects, and the patient's cognitive recognition of her perineal muscular activity.

The diagnosis of vaginismus is made during evaluation of the perineal body and distal vagina. In these patients, there is involuntary contraction of the pubococcygeus and levator sling. The patient does not realize it is present, nor is she (or you) able to overcome that contraction which persists as long as the attempt to examine continues. In severe cases, intravaginal examination is impossible without trauma.

The integrity of the perineal spinal reflex arc requires confirmation during the pelvic exam. The bulbocavernosus reflex, obtained by gently squeezing the clitoral glans with resultant contraction of the anal sphincter, demonstrates this adequately. If a component of the patients' complaint is the inability to feel anything, or anesthesia of certain vulvar areas, pain-pressure discrimination of the external genitals can evaluate sensory adequacy.

Vaginal Examination and Use of the Speculum

This immediately follows the external genital examination. After appropriately advising the patient, insert one finger into the introitus. Press on the perineal body and ask the patient to relax those muscles. In an apprehensive patient, instructions to first contract and then relax will effect the desired relaxation. Again advise the patient and insert a second finger, repeating perineal relaxation to obtain adequate introital diameter for speculum insertion. Vaginal speculae should be warm and moistened with tap water prior to insertion. The speculum is placed horizontally on the two fingers within the vagina and advanced while the vaginal fingers depress the perineal body. Once the first 1 to 2 cm. of the speculum have entered, the vaginal fingers are removed. For apprehensive patients, touching the thigh, mons, and external genitals before the vaginal introitus will avoid a startle-withdrawal response. Be careful that the speculum does not come into contact with the urethral meatus, as this is invariably painful. Warn patients about pressure sensations from the advancement and manipulation of the speculum.

Once the cervix is visualized, a pap smear from the squamo-columnar junction of the endocervical canal is made. The slide must be immediately placed in fixative for cytological reliability. Endocervical cultures for Neisseria gonorrhea are appropriately done routinely. Vaginal cultures are done on all patients with symptoms or evidence of vaginitis and include smear and culture techniques for bacteria, flagellates, and *Candida albicans.* In patients who complain of introital dyspareunia and vaginal burning following coitus, low-grade Candida and trichomonas infections are often found.

Cervical lacerations and scars can be significant in the etiology of deep thrust dyspareunia. Cervicitis is not associated with sexual dysfunction other than secondarily from irritative vulvo-vaginal symptoms. It does require treatment, however, for medical reasons.

The final portion of the speculum examination is withdrawal of the instrument while it remains partially open. In this way visualization is made of the entire vaginal mucosa with identification of possible pathological conditions.

Bimanual Examination

This procedure usually consists of two parts. First is the abdominal-vaginal, and second is the abdominal-recto-vaginal examination. For the first, two well-lubricated fingers are inserted into the vagina, one on either side of the cervix, and the other hand is used to depress the lower abdominal muscles. Assessment of uterine parameters, pain with movement of the cervix and uterus or point tenderness, and of each adnexa (including ovaries, fallopian tubes, and broad ligaments) can be made. Adequate evaluation of the posterior pelvis cannot be done without the abdominal recto-vaginal examination. For this, the patient is instructed to bear down and cautioned that she will feel the urge to defecate. One well-lubricated finger is inserted into the vagina and simultaneously one into the rectum. She is then instructed to relax. The recto-vaginal septum, posterior aspect of the uterus, posteriorly positioned ovaries or masses, and the utero-sacral ligaments can be assessed.

Proper use of the abdominal hand requires that the abdominal wall be depressed with that hand and pelvic structures then swept up against it with the vaginal fingers. It may be necessary to move that hand to five or six areas, but the initiation of vaginal and abdominal pressure is never simultaneous. Similarly, the fingers of the abdominal hand move as a unit, not separately. It produces an unpleasant experience for the patient, and additionally an unproductive clinical examination.

It is particularly important during the bimanual examination that the patient be aware of your movements and the sensations she will have. Her anxieties will be maximal because you have, in effect, invaded her vagina and pelvis with a portion of your body. Much of this will be allayed by your earlier approach to her, but unless care is taken during this last portion of the exam you will not gain potentially important information and she will remember the entire process as unpleasant. Be extremely cautious in considering the woman's reactions as a painful response. Elicit information which differentiates pressure, sensation of movement, urge to defecate, and urge to urinate which are always normally present in the bimanual examination. Compression of the ovary by bimanual entrapment always elicits pain just as compression of the testes does. It does not indicate pathology unless exquisite, or the ovary is noted to be in a fixed position from which it cannot move.

Many gynecological pathological entities exist which are etiological or contributory to sexual dysfunction. These require surgical or medical management followed by reevaluation and treatment of any remaining dysfunction. Do not assume that dysfunction that was primarily organic—for example, chronic pelvic infection—will disappear once the condition is corrected. Pain, fear, and inhibition may persist and require relearning and therapy before remission occurs.

EDUCATION IN SELF-AWARENESS

Familiarity with her own body is every woman's right and is often the first step in the sexual therapeutic process. Women should be encouraged and instructed in visual and tactile examination of their external genitals through use of a mirror. Self-exploration of the vagina and palpation of the cervix should ideally also be taught. Many women have felt restricted from this. Self-ignorance aggravates the problems of gynecological and sexual health. The physician's authority can remove at least some of this restriction. All women, at some point, must have evaluation by those competent to make full evaluation and to manage pathology. You provide that service for which she does not at this time have a tenable alternative.

chapter

11

For many couples the last months of pregnancy, and the early months postpartum, are sexually "off limits." Fears of infection or injury to the fetus, physical discomfort resulting from the changing female contour, and a negative female body image limit or disrupt sexuality. Is this cessation necessary? Does significant danger to the fetus exist from intercourse? Does abdominal distention preclude comfortable sexual positioning? What should we advise patients? Factually based, reasonable guidelines can be formulated for the late pregnancy and early postpartum couple.

Editor

Sexuality During Pregnancy and Postpartum

JULIUS C. BUTLER, M.D.

NATHANIEL N. WAGNER, Ph.D.

Despite the obvious importance of sexual activity during pregnancy, there is a remarkable lack of objective data about how people deal with their sexual needs during this time. For many people it is a time of stress. Therefore, the lack of scientific information is all the more remarkable as physicians are often asked for advice concerning sexuality during pregnancy.

As of early 1974 there were only three published studies which supply detailed normative data. One of these is the 1966 work of Masters and Johnson on human sexual response. The other two (Solberg *et al*; Falicov) were published in 1973. These studies shall be detailed later; first we will look at the reasons for the sparseness of information and the way in which practitioners have filled this void.

Physician Attitudes

Clearly, the most important reason for the avoidance of this area lies in the attitude that society holds toward sexuality. The medical world has accurately reflected the societal view which has considerable trouble in accepting sexuality and pregnancy at the same time in the same person. Whether the impending motherhood of the pregnant woman raises unconscious resistances in the physician (usually male) by mixing the unmixables, lover and mother, is one speculation.

Another important factor is the biological reality that in the vast majority of mammals sexual activity *does not* occur during the period of pregnancy. Only when the phylogenetic scale is ascended to the level of primates does sexual behavior during pregnancy occur. Even in primates, the pregnant female does not seek intercourse, but under pressure from the male, and when unable to move away from his attentions, will submit. This is not the case for human females, as we shall see when we look at the data.

A third reason for the lack of solid information, until rather recently, can be found in the youth of obstetrics and gynecology as a specialty. The American Board of Obstetrics and Gynecology was incorporated in 1930 while the American Medical Association dates to 1847. Until comparatively recent times, childbirth management was the province of the midwife. Midwifery flourished in Europe in the 17th, 18th, and 19th centuries. The physician, almost invariably male, was utilized only in the most serious circumstances. Indeed, the doctor rarely involved himself in what was "not quite proper medicine." One important resistance appeared to be the public horror at the indecency of exposure of the female.

In the United States, the general practitioner gradually became involved in the care of pregnant women. His initial involvement was a reluctant one and grew out of the fact that maternal mortality was a great burden for a fast growing and expanding nation. As medical skills and record keeping improved, maternal mortality and perinatal mortality demanded greater involvement of physicians. There was more and more resistance to home deliveries and insistence on the safe support of the hospital by the physician.

In all the growing involvement of physicians in pregnancy and childbirth, the focus was on reducing maternal and infant mortality. It was very scientific, very proper, and had nothing to do with sex, except in a distant way that was understood, but not talked about. Intercourse was not scientific and not a proper object of study.

Survey of Obstetrical Textbooks

A survey of the major textbooks in Obstetrics and Gynecology demonstrates that even today intercourse during pregnancy is treated in a hasty and superficial way. In an otherwise excellent text, *Synopsis of Obstetrics* (McLennan, 1970), coitus is only mentioned in relation to multiple pregnancy. The authors state that, due to the tendency toward premature labor, certain precautions should be observed, such as avoidance of coitus in the last 3 months, additional rest, and minimal travel. Similarly, Ried *et al.* in their textbook (1972) state that sexual intercourse is permitted through the seventh month of pregnancy, but should be curtailed at this time because of possible intrauterine infection, should the patient enter labor after intercourse. Willson, in *On the Management of Obstetrical Difficulties* (1961), lists under prenatal instructions "intercourse." He recommends that patients in whom previous abortions have occurred, or those with threatened abortions, should avoid intercourse during the first half of pregnancy. For other women, coitus is judged to be harmless until about 4 weeks before term, after which abstinence is recommended.

There is no general agreement on the length of time during pregnancy that intercourse may safely be practiced and when it should be discontinued. Many authorities imply that intercourse should be discontinued after the seventh month, while others state that coitus should be stopped 6 weeks before term. No author states clearly the data base or source of information from which these recommendations flow. It would appear that many physicians, fearing the potential contamination of the vaginal tract and subsequent intrauterine infection, feel that these risks would be minimized if coitus were interdicted in the later stages of pregnancy. Although this may have represented sound medical thought in the preantibiotic era, it is questionable today. It may well be that the feeling of inappropriateness of intercourse late in pregnancy was fostered in medical teachings, not so much from the desire to diminish maternal infection but as an expression of a societal taboo.

In the obstetrical text of Beck and Rosenthal (1975) the authors state that sexual intercourse may cause a miscarriage in the early months or premature labor in the later part of pregnancy, and in the event that either of these accidents occur the risks of infection are greatly increased. Restrictions are recommended with abstinence during the last 2 months. If at any time interruption of the pregnancy is threatened, coitus should be avoided throughout the remainder of gestation. They also list as possible causes of premature labor a fall or blow on the abdomen, running up and down stairs, long auto journeys, excessive vomiting, convulsions, horseback riding, golf, tennis, and excessive coitus. We are unable to ascertain the basis for this list.

These texts generally pay little attention to the possible relationship of coitus to abruptio placenta, habitual or threatened miscarriage, placenta previa, or premature labor.

It is not surprising, therefore, that physicians have not routinely asked about the following points while taking an obstetrical history: the frequency of coitus, the relative frequency of orgasm, personal satisfaction in sexual activity during pregnancy, self-perception (image-change), preferred positions of coitus, noncoital sex play, masturbatory practices, or the state of the male-female relationship. Even if this information were obtained by a physician, there would be difficulty utilizing it effectively.

Normative Studies

The first detailed study of sexual activity during pregnancy was part of the pioneering work of William H. Masters an obstetrician-gynecologist, and Virginia Johnson, a psychologist (1966). They studied 101 multiparas and primiparas and reported an initial decrease in coital desire and frequency in the first trimester. During the second trimester there was some increase in sexual interest and performance that they associated with increased congestion of the pelvic vasculature. The last trimester evidenced the most major drop in sexual interest and activity. Almost one-half of their sample reported continued low levels of sexuality at 3 months after delivery.

Solberg *et al.* (1973) interviewed 260 women in the immediate postpartum period. Only women having access to a sexual partner for at least 7 out of the 9 months of pregnancy were included in this sample. Because of this requirement, 98% of the sample was married.

Each woman was interviewed by one of three trained male medical-student interviewers while in the hospital on the second or third postpartum day. All women were aware of the nature and subject matter of the study; 15% of those asked refused to participate, and less than 1% discontinued the interview once begun. Of those refusing to participate, the median age was 26.6 years (identical with that of the sample). The racial background and religious preference of those refusing to participate did not differ significantly from the sample except that Asian-Americans had a higher refusal rate.

The most striking finding was the steady and consistent decrease in sexual activity during pregnancy for the majority of the subjects. Surprisingly, age, length of marriage, educational level, and other similar indicators were not associated with the decrease in sexual behavior. Stated level of sexual interest was the only factor correlated with behavior. Only in the last month of pregnancy was there no significant relationship between sexual interest and activity.

Orgasmic Function

Orgasmic activity during pregnancy was discussed with each woman. Only 7% reported never having experienced orgasm. Another 9% claimed orgasmic experience, although, by their description of orgasm, the interviewer thought they might be confusing orgasm with the excitement which is part of the plateau phase described by Masters and Johnson. Since these women did not differ significantly from other orgasmic women in social or behavioral data, they were included as orgasmic. Further, the experience of orgasm is a personal, internal one, and it is a questionable practice for someone to judge the internal experience of another.

As with intercourse, the percentage of coital acts leading to orgasm decreased as pregnancy progressed. In addition, there was a general decrease in the strength or intensity of orgasm compared to orgasmic intensity before pregnancy. It is noteworthy, however, that a small percentage of women consistently reported an increase in orgasmic intensity at all stages of pregnancy.

Other Sexual Behavior

Masturbation as an attempt to achieve orgasm had been used in the 2 years before pregnancy by 16% of the 260 women. Of these, approximately two-thirds had achieved orgasm by masturbation. Although some women continued to masturbate during pregnancy, the majority of the 16% did not. For those who continued to masturbate, the orgasmic rate with masturbation did not change significantly during pregnancy.

Hand stimulation by the woman's partner as an attempt to reach orgasm was used in the previous 2 years before pregnancy by 45% of the 260; of these, 118, (57%) has been successfully orgasmic at least once. Sixty percent of the women continued this activity during pregnancy. Orgasmic rate from hand stimulation did not seem to vary significantly during pregnancy.

Oral-genital stimulation in an attempt to reach orgasm was used by 39% of 257 women in the previous 2 years. Of these 99 women, fellatio was usually performed by 32%, and cunnilingus by 17%, while 50% used both with equal frequency or simultaneously. With oral-genital stimulation, 53% of the 99 women had been successful in reaching orgasm at least once. There were no significant differences between these three methods in terms of rate of use throughout pregnancy. Of the 99 using oral-genital stimulation to achieve orgasm, 42 to 55% did not use it during pregnancy. Orgasmic rates from oral-genital stimulation decline with pregnancy, from 16% reporting orgasm rarely or never prior to pregnancy to 58% in stage 9.

Only five women (2%) received recommendations from their physicians or other paramedical personnel concerning sexual activities that might be substituted for coitus in pregnancy. Hand stimulation was the activity recommended to satisfy both partners.

Coital Positions

The most impressive finding concerning coital positions was the decrease in the male superior position which has been used by these couples approximately 80% of the time. The side-by-side position became the most frequent in the last trimester and the rear entry position, which was rarely used prior to pregnancy, became much more popular.

There was no striking association between coital frequency and positions used, but there was a consistent, low-order relation, with more active women tending to use a side-by-side position in the last trimester more frequently than women of low sexual activity. There was no association between position used and orgasmic rate.

Of the 260 women, 10% received recommendations from their physicians or other paramedical personnel about positions that might be more comfortable in pregnancy. Side-by-side or rear entry was recommended to 5%, the rest receiving other recommendations.

Reasons for Change

Women reporting a change in degree or intensity of their sexual experience during pregnancy were questioned about the reason (or reasons) in their own minds for the change. Their responses, as grouped by the interviewers, were as follows: physical discomfort, 46%; fear of injury to the baby, 27%; loss of interest, 23%; awkwardness while having coitus, 17%; recommendation of physician, 8%; reasons extraneous to pregnancy, 6%; loss of attractiveness in woman's own mind, 4%; recommendation of person other than physician, 1%; and other reasons, 15%. The major reason for change, if more than one reason was given, followed the same distribution.

Of 260 women, 29% received instructions from their physicians recommending coital abstention, beginning at times ranging from 2 to 8 weeks before the estimated date of confinement. Women receiving such instructions were more likely to abstain from coitus in the last month. Other months showed no such relation.

Sexual Adjustment during First Pregnancy and Postpartum

The third normative study detailed the sexual adjustment of 19 primigravidas (Falicov, 1973). It was in striking agreement with the study noted above. Sexual patterns were evaluated postpartum. At 7 months the frequency of coitus and general sexuality was still depressed from prepregnancy levels. The investigator felt this was primarily the result of fatigue and psychological tensions from caring for the child, as sexual desire and eroticism had returned to normal or heightened level. In fact, a majority of the sample reported their capacity for arousal and orgasm to be greater than prior to pregnancy.

Discussion of Normative Studies

All three studies agree on a decline in sexual interest and activity in the first and third trimester. Masters and Johnson reported an increase in the second trimester. The third study, however, reported the decline in the second trimester not to be as sharp as during the first trimester. It has been suggested that the volunteer quality of the Masters and Johnson population may have biased their populations toward individuals with a particular interest in sexuality.

To what extent sexual response during pregnancy is directly responsive to hormonal, metabolic, or physical changes cannot now be answered. All three studies are in agreement that the women's response to pregnancy is highly variable with a minority experiencing greater sexual desire during pregnancy than experienced prior to pregnancy. Generally, however, there is a loss of sexual desire which becomes of greater magnitude as the pregnancy progresses.

The loss of sexual interest and desire is reflected in both coital and noncoital sexual behavior. The decrease in noncoital behavior, such as mutual oral-genital stimulation, strongly suggests that more than attitudes and comfort with sexuality is involved. Individuals who engage in mutual oral-genital stimulation are generally reasonably comfortable in accepting their sexuality. Furthermore, fear of penile penetration damaging the fetus would play no part in the reduction of this behavior. How much simple physical fatigue is at issue, and how much is hormonal or metabolic, must wait upon more sophisticated research.

It is clear that the human female undergoes a complicated series of physical, hormonal, and psychological changes during pregnancy. The response to these changes is quite variable, reflecting the highly individualistic nature of human sexuality and response to pregnancy.

Relationship to Premature Labor

One of the major reasons cited for discontinuing coitus is the fear of harm to the fetus either by infection or by bringing on labor prematurely. In fact, some investigations (Javert, 1957; Pugh and Fernandez, 1953) have argued that spontaneous abortion may be directly related to coitus during pregnancy. Although the authors do not support their hypothesis by experimental data, they argue their case cogently and the matter is clearly not settled.

The earliest study to look at the effects of coitus in late pregnancy was that of Pugh and Fernandez. They studied 500 women and concluded that coitus was not responsible for the various complications of late pregnancy, delivery, and the puerperium frequently attributed to it. Similarly, our study found no relationship between coital activity and prematurity. Out of 260 women, none had noticed the immediate onset of labor after coitus or orgasm. Birthweight, gestational age at delivery and Apgar scores at 1 min. were all independent of coitus and rate of orgasm in the last trimester.

Orgasm and Premature Labor

There has been interesting speculation and experimental work suggesting that coitus *per se* may not be related to premature labor, but that orgasm may (Javert, 1957; Linner, 1969). One of the most vocal proponents of this view is Goodlin (1969) who has supplied clinical data in support of this relationship. In another paper Goodlin *et al.* (1971*b*) reported on the fetal heart rates and uterine tension during maternal orgasm, induced by masturbation in a gravida at term. Associated uterine contractions and deceleration of fetal heart rate were noted in the single case. In a letter in the New England Journal of Medicine discussing the findings of the Seattle study, however, Goodlin wrote he may have overstated his case to make a point he felt to be very important. This issue is not yet resolved.

Uterine Contractions

The possible relationship of orgasm to premature delivery might be through the mechanism of induced uterine contractions. Masters and Johnson have demonstrated the existence of uterine contractions during orgasm. They have also commented on the similarity of uterine contractions in orgasm to the contractions of labor. Anecdotal experience of the authors reinforces the similarities of contractions in these two conditions. A patient of one of the authors described her second delivery without anesthesia as "the biggest orgasm" she had ever experienced.

This view receives some support from the Seattle study in a separate report (Wagner *et al.*, 1974) which found a relationship between prematurity and multiple orgasm during pregnancy. The numbers involved were small and the authors, while feeling there may, in fact, be a relationship between prematurity and multiple orgasm, state that more research is needed before definitive conclusions can be drawn.

Prostaglandins

There is one further way in which coitus might possibly be related to premature labor. Prostaglandins, a group of fatty acid derivatives present in human semen, have definitely been associated with uterine contractions. In fact, there has been considerable experimental work using prostaglandins as a method of inducing abortions. At the present time, however, there is no real evidence linking prostaglandins in human semen with premature labor, nor is there the kind of evidence that can rule out an association. A careful study of the factors associated with premature labor left a large percentage unexplained. Adam (1959), in a survey of factors in premature labor lists 43% of 1,186 premature labors as essentially unexplained.

In summary, the relationship of coitus and orgasm to premature labor is presently unclear. Although there are some suggestive relationships and some suggestive findings, the two studies that look at reasonably large samples of pregnant women found no relationship between coitus during pregnancy and premature labor.

Counseling the Pregnant Couple

How should the physician deal with the pregnant patient and her partner concerning their sexual activity during pregnancy? First, the involvement of the male must be viewed as important. Traditionally, physicians have only dealt with the female, leaving her anxiety about sexuality and her concerns about her partner to be handled by herself. Many women fear that during pregnancy, when she may see herself as unattractive and "unsexy," the partner will seek sexual gratification elsewhere. During pregnancy, many women need additional support and closeness from their men. Because of these factors, it is essential that the physician attempt to understand the male-female relationship and provide help where it is needed.

Potential Dangers of Coitus during Pregnancy

It is useful to think of the potential dangers of coitus during pregnancy in three main areas: 1) mechanical, 2) infection, and 3) uterine contractions. (Neubardt, 1973).

Mechanical. The main fear is related to the possible damage caused by the penis during coital thrusting. Possible deleterious effects could be ruptured membranes, amniotitis, or placental bleeding. Our survey of the literature and the experience of the senior author provide no support for these potential hazards. Naturally, bleeding is a serious symptom that during the third trimester might indicate plancenta previa. Any substantial bleeding is clearly a contraindication to intercourse until the source of the bleeding is diagnosed and the matter satisfactorily managed.

Infection. During active coitus the penis can encourage the migration of vaginal bacteria into the upper genital organs. This represents a threat to the woman with an incompetent cervical os, ruptured membranes, or an effaced or dilated cervix late in gestation. A competent cervix and intact membranes provide perfectly adequate protection against infection for the healthy pregnant woman.

Uterine Contractions. There is no question that orgasm may produce uterine contractions. Obviously, this can present a problem to the habitual aborter, the woman who is threatening to abort, or the woman who may enter premature labor. Since there may not be any sure way to determine who may enter premature labor, it appears sensible to recommend limitations on coitus to women who have previously delivered prematurely or who are found on vaginal examination to have a dilated cervix or any finding suggesting either premature labor or an unusually small fetus.

All women should be given the information that orgasm might bring on labor late in pregnancy. The key factor is orgasm, and therefore, noncoital activity leading to orgasm should be considered synonymous with coitus leading to orgasm. Sexual behavior, both coital and noncoital, not leading to orgasm, need not be limited, as there seems no relationship to uterine contractions.

Positions during Coitus

For those couples who want to continue coital behavior, it is important for the physician to provide specific assistance about coital techniques. Early in pregnancy, the positions favored by the couple can be maintained. As pregnancy progresses, most couples find the side-by-side and rear entry positions to be most comfortable and enjoyable.

Late in pregnancy (34 to 38 weeks) the fetal head will often become engaged. Coitus in these circumstances will produce vaginal and abdominal discomfort and may alarm both partners. Here, and in other circumstances, the physician can recommend noncoital activity for those couples who want to continue sexual activity. The primacy of coitus, biologically and historically, is based on the relationship of coitus to conception. The pregnant couple need not be tied to coitus as the only or primary method of sexual activity.

The Postpartum Response

The couple often wonder when coital behavior can be resumed after delivery. Obviously noncoital behavior such as fondling and petting can be resumed immediately, or as soon as the female is interested. Sexual interest in the woman will probably be low in the immediate postpartum period. The return of sexual interest is highly variable. The physician should encourage the couple to resume their customary level and type of sexual activity as soon as they wish. If bleeding or discomfort because of the episiotomy rule out early coital behavior, other noncoital behavior will ease this time and the resumption to prepregnancy levels and activities.

A Cautionary Note

Noncoital activities have been generally encouraged in this chapter as a method of continuing sexual communication when there is some reason to limit or abstain from coitus. There is, however, a sexual practice with clear danger to the pregnant female. One of the infrequently practiced methods of cunnilingus consists of the male forcing air into the vagina. Some women report high excitement and even orgasm with this technique. For pregnant women, this unusual method of cunnilingus provides risk. Aronson (1969), writing from the Medical Examiner's office in Philadelphia, has reported a number of cases where death has followed the forceful insufflation of the vagina with air. The individuals who died were uniformly found to have intravascular gas. In each instance, death was due to an air embolism. Findings on autopsy have demonstrated entrance by the endocervical canal (generally dilated by 1 to 1.5 cm) into the maternal vascular system. Aronson also found cases previously reported in America, England, and Germany.

This chapter has reviewed the relationship of sexual behavior to pregnancy. Physician attitudes were discussed as the major reason for the prevalence of variety of unsubstantiated beliefs about this topic. Major research findings indicate a decrease in sexual interest and activity throughout pregnancy. Although this was true for the majority of women studied, for some women sexual interest was enhanced by pregnancy. The response to pregnancy is highly individualistic and the decrease or increase in sexual interest and activity is not predictable by socioeconomic or demographic factors.

Data also exist with respect to the possible relationship of coitus and orgasm to premature labor. Based on these facts, recommendations concerning counseling can be made. Physicians have a responsibility to provide assistance to patients and their mates in this time which is unnecessarily stressful to many people.

REFERENCES

Adam, G. S. 1959. Aetiological Factors in Premature Labour, J. Obstet. Gynecol. 66: 732-736.

Aronson, M. 1969. Fatal Air Embolism Caused by Bizarre Sexual Behavior during Pregnancy. Med. Aspects Human Sexuality. December. 33-39.

Beck, A. C. and Rosenthal, A. H. 1975. *Obstetrical Practice.* 7th Ed. pp. 245, 907. Baltimore: Williams & Wilkins.

Falicov, C. J. 1973. Sexual Adjustment during First Pregnancy and Postpartum. Am. J. Obstet. Gynecol. 117: 991-1000.

Goodlin, R. C. 1969. Orgasm and Premature Labour. Lancet, 2: 646.

Goodlin, R. C., Keller, D. W., and Raffin, M. 1971a. Orgasm during Late Pregnancy: Possible Deleterious Effects. Obstet. Gynecol. 38: 916-920.

Goodlin, R. C. Schmidt, W., and Creevy, D. C. 1971b. Uterine Tension and Fetal Heart Rate during Maternal Orgasm. Obstet. Gynecol. 39: 125-127.

Javert, C. T. 1957. *Spontaneous and Habitual Abortion.* New York: McGraw-Hill.

Linner, R. R. 1969. *Sex and the Unborn Child.* New York: Julian Press.

Masters, W. H. and Johnson, V. E. 1966. *Human Sexual Response.* Boston: Little Brown.

McLennan, C. E., 1970 *Synopsis of Obstetrics.* 8th ed. p. 212. St. Louis: Mosby.

Neubardt, S. 1973. Coitus During Pregnancy. Med. Aspects Human Sexuality. September. 197-198.

Pugh, W. E. and Fernandez, F. L. 1953. Coitus in Late Pregnancy: A Follow-up Study of the effects of Coitus on Late Pregnancy, Delivery and the Puerperium. Obstet. Gynecol. 2: 636-642.

Reid, D. E., Ryan, K. J. and Benirschke, K. 1972. *Principles and Management of Human Reproduction.* Philadelphia: Saunders.

Solberg, D. A., Butler, J., and Wagner, N. N. 1973. Sexual Behavior in Pregnancy. N. Eng. J. Med. 288: 1098-1103.

Wagner, N. N., Butler, J. C., and Sanders, J. 1974. Prematurity and Sexual Activity during Pregnancy. To be published.

Willson, J. R., 1961. *On the Management of Obstetrical Difficulties. p. 80. St. Louis: Mosby.*

chapter

12

For most lay persons and many physicians, the reaction to seeing a person in a wheel chair includes the assumption that he or she must have no sex life. Perhaps this myth has been perpetuated by popular novels like Lady Chatterly's Lover, *in which the lady, sexually frustrated in consequence of her husband's paralysis, turns to another man. Perhaps the attitude has been perpetuated in medicine by the knowledge that sensory loss occurs with complete spinal transection and that interruption of brain-penis circuitry precludes erectile response to sexual thought. Beyond this, concerns over bladder and bowel emptying have compounded the patients' reticence to broach what they anticipate as yet another devastating topic.*

Spinal cord injury patients are of increasing medical significance. High speed automobile and motorcycle crashes, surf board accidents, civilian gunshot wounds, and the victims of international warfare contribute inexorably to their rising number.

What styles of sexual expression are available to these patients? Patients have the right to this knowledge. Physicians have the responsibility to present that knowledge. But first, they *must know.*

Editor

Sexuality and the Spinal Cord Injured

THEODORE *M*. COLE, *M*.D.

When considerations of human sexuality and physical disability combine in the same individual they significantly effect the doctor-patient relationship. The possibility of errors in clinical judgment and procedure are doubled because taboos and misinformation surround the area of physical disability as well as the area of sexuality.

Medical student textbooks have generally been silent on the subject of physical disability and sexuality. Patients with physical disabilities may be seen by physicians in general practice or in any one of the specialty practices. They are often seen by specialists in Rehabilitation Medicine, a relatively new specialty. Rehabilitation Medicine is "a treatment process designed to help physically handicapped individuals make maximal use of residual capacities and to enable them to obtain optimal satisfaction and usefulness in terms of themselves, their families, and their community" (Krusen *et al.,* 1971). Rehabilitation, therefore, concerns itself with the treatment of the entire patient rather than a sequestered portion of anatomy or physiology. The involvement is often so comprehensive as to require participation by an entire team of medical and paramedical professionals. Yet a textbook for medical students, published in 1971 and dealing exclusively with rehabilitation of the physically disabled, includes human sexuality on only two of 892 pages.

A review of seven textbooks on sex education for medical students yields a total of 27 pages which deal with the effect of trauma, surgery, and physical handicaps upon human sexual expression. More optimistically, however, a

147

recent text on management of the arthritic patient devoted approximately 10% to the discussion of sexual aspects of arthritis (Ehrlich, 1973).

IMPORTANCE OF SEXUALITY OF THE PHYSICALLY DISABLED

As much as 10% of the adult population in the United States today has a physical handicap which in some way poses a substantial limitation to normal activities (Finley, 1972). Examples include arthritis, stroke, heart disease, end stage renal disease, amputations, deformities, visual or auditory impairment, disfiguring scars, paralysis, and developmental anomalies. On a humanitarian basis alone the sexuality of physically disabled people should not be forgotten. When given a chance to speak for themselves, people with physical disabilities underscore the importance of their sexuality and their libidinous drives which may be unaltered by their physical disabilities (Richardson, 1972). Weiss and Diamond (1966), studying a group of adults with spinal cord disease, found that they tended to avoid a realistic and conscious consideration of their sexuality at the same time that they exhibited a similar avoidance of realistic acceptance of their disabilities. This may be of special importance since the successful rehabilitation outcome may be totally frustrated by the patient's inability to consider and integrate his altered self or to build a new life based upon reality rather than unrealistic hopes. Hopefully, as the clinician becomes more comfortable working with the patient's realistic sexual expectations, he or she may discover that sexuality is a potent tool in facilitating reality acceptance in general.

MYTHS

The myths and emotions that surround human sexuality are compounded by the myths and emotions that are attached to such words as crippled, handicapped, paralyzed, maimed, or deformed. As is true for other myths, those that grow out of the area of physical disability are both old and contradictory. In 1588 Michael deMontaigne, in his essay, "Of Cripples," wrote, "...they say...that he does not know venus in her perfect sweetness who has not lain with a cripple... ." The rationale for this notion is that the lame woman's energies, not being expended for ambulation, have been preserved for sexual activity. Nutrition and vigor which are denied to the lame legs are channeled instead to the genitals which become fuller, better nourished, and more vigorous (Benedick, 1971).

There are common misconceptions that physically disabled people do not feel a need for sexual expression or that sex is not important to them. Oftentimes it is believed that the paralyzed or deformed person is not able to engage in sexual intercourse at all. Disabled people frequently are thought to have foul odors associated with their bodies. There is a frequent stereotypic association of mental retardation with conspicuous physical disability. Indeed, there is a certain hostility toward the handicapped that appears as eugenicist notions of segregating or disposing of disabled people in order not to weaken the able-bodied stock.

Many able-bodied people are repulsed by adults with physical disabilities. In addition, some fear that the physically disabled will breed more disability. The fear may be of genetic transmission or that the disabled adult will not be able to rear a mentally healthy child because of the limitations imposed upon the parent role by the physical disability.

Conversely, some myths and misconceptions surrounding physical disability and sexuality attach excessive if not perverse sexual desires and capabilities on to the disabled person. Children's fairy tale books have traditionally depicted the villain in the form of an ugly troll who waits under the bridge for unsuspecting travelers. For some able-bodied people there is the fear that the physically disabled may surpass them in sexual capabilities. This notion is especially difficult to integrate with the paternalism which the able-bodied majority of society frequently shows toward its disabled counterparts. The condescending and paternalistic attitudes may manifest themselves in the ideas that the disabled person should appreciate anything we give him and that he has no right to be selective, seductive, or competitive. The end result is that the able-bodied majority has created a physical and emotional societal structure which imposes barriers to successful travel, communication, and adult experience.

Many of these myths are reinforced in the medical and educational literature. Money (1967) states that "the patient's index on the popularity parade ...is at the bottom of the list...paraplegia is sexually totally disabling." Herman (1950) studied 19 paraplegic male patients and concluded that the loss of somesthetic stimuli from the genital organs is primarily responsible for what he considers to be the absence of sexual excitation. He believed that sexual excitation was reduced because some of his subjects denied that they experienced sexual excitation after injury. This is in contrast with our experience and should raise the question of whether his subjects were denying sexual excitation in response to the researcher's own denial of their sexuality, or denying their sexuality as a defense against the psychological shock of traumatic paralysis. Stating that sex education for cerebral palsied children must be different from sex education for able-bodied children, Fox (1971) degrades the role and importance of sexual fantasy. Since sex is a bodily experience, he believes that physical joy is expressed through bodies, not minds, and that sex in the head "titillates without fulfilling." The body of the handicapped person, therefore, is scarcely something that gives pleasure. He suggests that sex education for such severely physically handicapped children should include emphasis upon sublimation as a substitution and commitment to an ideal such as religion.

Evidence accumulates, however, that the disabled person does not believe these myths. Cole *et al.* (1973) reported on a series of group discussions about sexuality with paraplegic and quadriplegic adult males and females. He had the opportunity to compare able-bodied single and married medical students and their partners with single and married spinal cord injured adults in a discussion seminar on human sexuality using identical movies to evoke discussion. He found that the disabled groups more quickly came to grips with meaningful discussion than the able-bodied medical students. There was less social chitchat among the disabled and fewer expressions of boredom, criticism, and annoyance with the movies and discussions. The disabled were ready and able to discuss their sexual concerns more openly and less defensively than the able-bodied groups. Of particular concern to them was the status of their ability to reproduce and their concern for self-image. The role of fantasy with this group was very strong. Many found personal physical satisfaction in satisfying their partners. Many reported that they used their partner's sensory experience to stimulate their own. Some complained about the protective, fatherly attitude of their attending physicians. One conclusion drawn from this work is that if any of the myths about sexuality and the spinal cord injured person have been dispelled, it is the myth that sex cannot or should not be discussed frankly with the physically disable person. In fact, the disabled demonstrated in many respects that they were capable of dealing with anxiety-producing material in a more direct and tolerant manner than many of the able-bodied people with whom they were compared.

CLASSIFICATION OF PHYSICAL DISABILITIES AND SEXUALITY

It is beyond the scope of this chapter to explore all of the physical impairments which may affect human sexual expression. However, it is useful to have a frame of reference for thinking about several physical disabilities and how they may affect human sexuality.

A simple but important point of separation of physical disabilities is their conspicuousness. Those which are conspicuous provide a continuing stimulus to be dealt with. Those which are inconspicuous can be kept from society, especially with regard to sexual implications. For example, male impotence may be known only to the man who is affected and his partner. Although he may be greatly concerned about his masculinity, he can conceal his concern from friends and acquaintances, even from people to whom he is sexually attracted, providing he avoids genital sexual activity. However, the disability of paraplegia is apparent for everyone to see. The paraplegic cannot delude himself. It is clear to him that most people wonder about him and his sexual adequacy. It has been our experience that those adults with conspicuous physical disabilities have had forced upon them an opportunity to think hard about their self-image and their sexual adequacy. Although some will seek comfort in a veneer or disinterest, bravado, machismo, or coquetry, most who have achieved satisfying sexual adjustment have dealt more honestly with themselves than their able-bodied counterparts.

Those disabilities which fall into the conspicuous group include brain injury, spinal cord injury, amputation, arthrogryposis, scoliosis, arthritis, blindness, deafness, dwarfism, and disfiguring scars. Inconspicuous disabilities that might affect sexuality include genital anomalies, disfigurements which are concealed by clothing, enterostomies, heart disease, diabetes mellitus, epilepsy, mastectomy, and surgical removal of pelvic organs.

A more detailed classification of physical disabilities, however, places disabilities into three groups separated by the time of onset of the disability and whether or not it is a static or progressive condition. Although it is not possible to classify every physical disability, it is possible to assess every patient from the point of view of functional impairment, thereby providing a framework for considering the effect of the disability upon sexuality and the therapeutic possibilities. For purposes of this classification it is assumed that the disabled person, when engaged in other than solitary sex activities, is doing so with an able-bodied or nearly able-bodied partner.

Type I: Physical Disabilities Acquired at Birth or in Early Childhood. This group includes brain injury, spinal cord disease or injury, skeletal amputations and deformities (especially hip joint disease preventing abduction of the hips and upper extremity amputation), altered body growth, heart disease, blindness, and deafness (Table 1).

Progressive congenital disabilities will not be considered here since few would permit the patient to survive past adolescence into adulthood when sexual activity would become an important consideration. The focus here is

TABLE 1

Symbols (♂, ♀) indicate for each sex the conspicuousness and the areas of sexual function which are often significantly affected by nonprogressive physical disabilities acquired in early life.

RELATIONSHIP OF PHYSICAL DISABILITY TO SEXUALITY

Type of disability: **Stable**
Time of onset: **Early Life, Prepuberty**

	Masturbation	Coitus	Fertility	Conspicuous to Society
Brain Injury				♂ ♀
Spinal Cord: Motor and Sensory loss	♂ ♀	♂	♂	♂ ♀
Skeletal: Amputation, Deformity	♂ ♀	♂♀		♂ ♀
Altered Body Growth				♂ ♀
Heart Disease				
Blindness				♂ ♀
Deafness				♂ ♀

upon those congenital disabilities which are nonprogressive and with which the patient can expect to live out a normal life expectancy.

Individuals with these disabilities have gone through childhood and adolescence as conspicuously different from their able-bodied counterparts. They have frequently been segregated from their peers and lack basic social skills. Although they may develop unusual abilities to read other people's feelings, these skills may be focused narcissistically upon their own needs.

In regard to social experience and marriage, a handicapped colleague has written, "If the child goes to a special school he sees only people like himself, which may have a channeling effect upon his dating. Grouping him with people like himself is often necessary if they are to participate in activities together and to mobilize necessary transportation. If the child goes to an ordinary school he is likely to be taken along in groups on school-sponsored events but not included in individual dating away from school.

"There are likely to be gaps in the handicapped person's experiences of daily living which may result in his inability to relate to other people. More importantly, he may miss social cues because he finds that he simply doesn't understand what's going on between people. He may also be intolerant of what may appear to be frivolity in his peer group, since life for him has been much more serious and purposeful with few things done just for the fun of it. Even those things that are done for fun may involve much effort from other people and he may question his right to demand it from others. An additional element may be that his peers regard him as a rather serious and dull person.

"Some of the experiential gaps can be overcome by reading, but no printed page can provide the feedback of facial expression for a blind person or even give the meaning of body language to a child who has had contact mainly with adults or other children too handicapped to employ body English. This is true of able-bodied people too, of course, if they go to a foreign country or fail to develop social maturity for some reason.

"One can see, therefore, that the handicapped person may have difficulty finding a compatible mate for marriage. Some of the subtleties of the search can easily escape recognition. The physically handicapped adult may find that he or she is more likely to be appealing to a mature individual who is there-fore likely to be older and have a greater chance of dying first and leaving the handicapped partner alone and once again in need of assistance. On the other hand, the compatible partner may himself have an excessive need to nurture. If this is met by a need for receiving nurturing on the part of the handicapped person, things may work out well provided there is no personality change in either partner as time goes on. If the chosen partner has neurotic reasons for marrying a handicapped person, the chances of a success are poor.

"Depending upon the degree of handicap, the honeymoon may be a dif-ficult time for handicapped people. Privacy may be hard to find if much physical assistance is needed. Traveling may be difficult to manage and access to public buildings may be difficult or impossible if help is not available. Careful planning may help to make a successful honeymoon possible but if it is unsuccessful, yet another aspect of life and marriage has been different or less than normal.

"A handicapped couple may be isolated in their own community if they are unable to relate to others and if they cannot participate in the activities of the community. The community may become afraid of them.

"Aging may place further stresses on the handicapped couple. This may be more marked than for the able-bodied partnership. Often the degree of handicap increases as loss of compensatory mechanisms increases with aging. In order to secure needed additional care, it may be necessary for the couple to be parted since most nursing homes and extended care facilities do not provide for accommodation of married couples, even able-bodied ones" (Easton, unpublished).

It is not difficult to see therefore, that the liabilities which some people carry into their sexual lives are there as if as a result of deliberate planning by society. Even if one can overcome the shyness to ask, it is uncommon for such a person to find understanding and informed sexual counseling. More often the informant is ignorant of the subject and too embarrassed to help anyway.

The net effect of these societal forces has often been to arrest or deflect the normal maturation process. This gives rise to an adult who often lacks some of the essential building blocks of the adult personality which society expects.

Table 1 also shows that congenital or early acquired heart disease is an example of a prepubescent physical disability which does not usually affect the maturation process nor stigmatize the individual with its conspicuousness. However, this disability does not generally affect sexual function.

Other disabilities may affect masturbation, ability to engage in coitus, or fertility. In addition, except for heart disease, they are all conspicuous to the casual observer. The impact upon sexuality of infertility or inability to engage in coitus is obvious. So too is the effect of limited masturbatory capability during and after puberty. This is important since masturbation is one way for the emerging adult to get in touch with his body.

Type II: Physical Disabilities Acquired Suddenly after Puberty, but Not Progressive: Since these conditions have their onset after the pubertal years, the maturation process has been completed and is therefore unaffected (Table 2). Many are conspicuous. Those which are covered by normal clothing are not. Examples include: spinal cord motor and sensory paralysis; spinal cord motor paralysis only; skeletal amputations and deformities (especially hip joint disease and upper extremity loss); genital injuries, amputations or removal of pelvic organs; disfiguring burns; enterostomies; blindness, and deafness.

Spinal cord injury is not only conspicuous but affects masturbation for both sexes and coitus and fertility for males. Skeletal amputations or deformities may affect masturbation and coitus in both sexes. Similarly, genital

TABLE 2

Symbols (♂, ♀) indicate for each sex the conspicuousness and the areas of sexual function which are often significantly affected by nonprogressive physical disabilities acquired suddenly after puberty.

RELATIONSHIP OF PHYSICAL DISABILITY TO SEXUALITY

Type of disability: **Suddenly acquired, Stable**
Time of onset: **Postpuberty**

	Masturbation	Coitus	Fertility	Conspicuous to Society
Spinal Cord : Motor and Sensory loss	♂ ♀	♂	♂	♂ ♀
Spinal Cord : Motor paralysis only	♂ ♀			♂ ♀
Skeletal : Amputation, Deformity	♂ ♀	♂ ♀		♂ ♀
Genital amputation, Deformity	♂ ♀	♂ ♀	♂	
Disfiguring injuries				♂ ♀
Enterostmy	♂ ♀	♂	♂	
Blindness				♂ ♀
Deafness				♂ ♀

injuries may affect masturbation and coitus in both sexes and fertility in the male. Disfiguring injuries, blindness, and deafness are most often notable only for their conspicuousness. Enterostomy may affect masturbation in both sexes and coitus and fertility in the male. Fertility would be affected in none of the females with sudden acquired postpubertal disabilities. All except genital injuries and enterostomies are conspicuous. Spinal cord injury is discussed in greater detail later.

Type III: Physical Disabilities Acquired after Puberty and Progressive. These conditions progress slowly and may lead to early death (Table 3). A particular characteristic of these disabilities is their effect upon the patient's sexual partner. The physician should be aware that intertwined with a sexual concern may be an underlying concern that sexual activity may accelerate the

TABLE 3

Symbols (♂, ♀) indicate for each sex the conspicuousness and the areas of sexual function which are often significantly affected by progressive physical disabilities acquired slowly after puberty.

RELATIONSHIP OF PHYSICAL DISABILITY TO SEXUALITY

Type of disability: Slowly acquired, Progressive
Time of onset: Postpuberty

	Masturbation	Coitus	Fertility	Conspicuous to Society
Heart Disease		♂♀		
Stroke				♂ ♀
Diabetes Mellitus	♂♀	♂	♂	
Muscular Dystrophy				♂♀
Multiple Sclerosis	♂♀	♂	♂	♂♀
Skeletal: Amputation, Deformity	♂♀	♂♀		♂♀
Renal Disease, end stage	♂♀	♂	♂	

course of the disease or even bring about a catastrophic episode such as death. These concerns may have an enormous impact upon the frequency and intensity of sexual activity and thus affect the relationship.

Conversely, progressive disabilities may have the opposite effect. The person may wish to fill out his sexual life now rather than risk losing out later. This may lead to a desperate attempt to include a series of sexual experiences which would otherwise have been left to more gradual inclusion, if at all.

A third possible concomitant of progressive disability is a deteriorating marital relationship. This may come about when there is virtually no opportunity for the couple to establish a stable relationship based upon a fixed physical condition. The couple is constantly adapting and adjusting to progressive losses which may overwhelm their ability to cope. Added to this is a generalized guilt which some able-bodied people report. The guilt may be found in either member of the partnership or it may affect concerned members of the family or close friends. There may be a strong pressure to desist from sexual activity because it is thought to be an unthinkable act to impose upon someone who is sick. This attitude overlooks the fact that many ill people choose to remain sexually interested and active to the extent that their illness will allow them.

End stage renal disease is one form of progressive disease which may affect sexuality and which has a special impact on the patient and partner. Many suffer not only from surgical interventions on their behalf but also from the metabolic consequences of electrolyte disturbance, uremia, anemia, and toxic neuropathy. As a result, fatigue, weight loss, anorexia, and impotence may result. Throughout the entire process the patient may become intensely aware of the importance of urinary output. The attention thus drawn to the genitals and urine may lend an additional twist to the emotional set which surrounds these organs. Or, the emotional set of the partner may be similarly affected. There may be a profound reluctance to use those same organs for physical pleasure in view of the illness and its medical concomitants.

As shown in Table 3, masturbation may be affected in both sexes by diabetes mellitus, multiple sclerosis, skeletal amputations and deformities, and end stage renal disease. Coitus may be affected for both sexes in heart disease and skeletal amputations and deformities, while it is more likely that only a male would be susceptible to losing his ability to engage in coitus as a result of diabetes mellitus, multiple sclerosis, and end stage renal disease. Additionally, the male's fertility may be affected in diabetes mellitus, multiple sclerosis, skeletal amputations and deformities, and end stage renal disease. Both sexes would be conspicuous in society with the disabilities of stroke, muscular dystrophy, multiple sclerosis, or skeletal amputations and deformities.

The treatment of any of the above conditions can affect sexuality. Medications used to treat some of these conditions can affect penile erection and ejaculation.

SPINAL CORD INJURY AND SEXUALITY

The effect of spinal cord injury upon sexuality deserves separate discussion. Improvements in the medical management of paraplegia and quadriplegia allow normal life expectancies after injury. Increased numbers of patients with this disability have been caused by recent wars and the hazards of an industrialized and mobile society. Spinal cord injured people have organized lobbies for more effective care by health professionals and have begun to demand counseling and assistance in the pursuit of sexual rehabilitation.

It is difficult for people unaccustomed to interacting with spinal injured adults to appreciate the impact of the obvious and subtle aspects of the disability. However, its effect upon sexuality can be better appreciated if the reader will imagine for a moment that he has suddenly become totally paralyzed and has lost sensation from the breasts down. Imagine that normal bowel and bladder control has been lost and that the bladder empties through a tube which travels down the leg to a plastic bag strapped to the calf and filled with yellow urine. In addition, voluntary control of the anal sphincter has been lost and fecal incontinence can occur without warning. The genitals have lost all cutaneous sensation. One would have to watch in order to know that they were being touched. Orgasm in the physical sense has been lost and for the male psychically controlled erections cannot occur in spite of intense arousal. Spasticity of the lower body is a daily phenomenon and periodic spasms of the legs may cause them to flex at the knees and hips or scissor together. Once rounded and full areas of the body are now replaced by bony prominences. There no longer remains the ability to stand and walk and the environment is viewed from about 4 ft. above the ground. Conversation is carried on with erect people by tilting back the head and looking up. Self-consciousness about one's own body may lead some to avoid sexual contact altogether. For others the alteration of the body is so profound as to call into question whether sexual expression can even remotely resemble previous sexual patterns.

As a result of myths and widespread ignorance, the physician should carefully set his expectations for the wide assortment of methods with which patients and hospital staff deal with sexual concerns. The most common is mutual silence or avoidance of sexual discussion. Another is limitation of discussion to procreation and fertility. Less commonly the physician and the patient may discuss intercourse simply as pleasure, recreation, and communication. It is even less common for the physician and the patient to discuss sexual options other than intercourse, including manual and oral-genital stimulation, the use of devices such as dildos and vibrators, and techniques of pleasuring. In our experience it is rare for the physician to instruct patients in the use of fantasy.

When paraplegic and quadriplegic patients feel permission, they may present the physician with a variety of challenging questions. "How do I have intercourse while wearing a urethral catheter? How do I manage hygienic problems associated with bowel and bladder incontinence? How can I have sex if I have an ileal conduit (an operation which diverts urine flow away from the bladder to a loop of intestine which exits at the abdominal wall into a plastic bag). What can I do about the severe headache I get when my genitals are stimulated? What positions can I use for sexual intercourse? What techniques can you teach me for having "quickies" when I have just a brief amount of time and not enough for transferring to a bed and undressing? How can I have sex without getting out of the wheelchair? Is my partner likely to become infected by having intercourse with me, since my urine is infected? Can I remove my catheter for sex and then replace it?"

Many of these questions require little more than common sense, open communication and a willingness to experiment. Women can tape the catheter to the thigh away from the vagina. Men can fold it down and along side the penis, pull a condom over it and the penis, and lubricate well. Sphincter incontinence requires adequate discussion with the partner before sex commences, then simply avoidance of those positions and stimuli that are known to precipitate bladder or bowel emptying. An ileal conduit urine collecting bag can be positioned out of the way to avoid chaffing which may break the seal. It is also helpful to keep a towel handy in case of accidents. The severe headaches are caused by hypertension secondary to autonomic hyperreflexia and sympathetic nervous system overactivity, which is evoked reflexly by pelvic organ stimulation. It is relieved immediately by stopping the stimulation briefly. Quick sexual contacts are generally accomplished in the wheel chair and often utilize oral-genital activity. Sexual intercourse can be experienced by the disabled male in his wheelchair with the female sitting on his lap with her back toward him. Urinary tract infections will almost never infect the partner when ordinary hygiene is observed. The catheter can be removed before sex and a new one replaced by sterile technique after completion of sexual activity (Mooney *et al.* In press).

MALE SEXUALITY AND SPINAL CORD INJURY

Most of the medical literature on paraplegia, quadriplegia, and human sexuality focuses on the act of sexual intercourse and its correlates. Zeitlin *et al.* (1957) reported on 100 cases of spinal cord injury. Fifty-four percent of the males could achieve penile erection and 26% could complete intercourse.

However, only 5% experienced orgasm and only 3% had ejaculations. Tsuji *et al.* (1961) studied 655 spinal injured adults and reported that 54% of the males were able to have penile erections. This rose to 80% 1 year after injury. Comarr (1970) studied 150 and reported that the overall incidence of psychogenically stimulated erections was 23%, while erections occurred spontaneously in 75% and could be mechanically stimulated in 71%. Of his patients, 38% attempted coitus, but 24% were unsuccessful. Another 38%, however, did not even attempt it. From Germany, Jochheim and Wahle reported (1970) on libido in a group of spastic and flaccid paraplegics. In the spastic group, libido or sexual drive, upon hospital discharge, was present in only 7.1% but increased to 26.1% after 1 year. In the flaccid group, none claimed libido at the time of discharge, but 5.6% reported sexual interest 1 year after discharge.

Reflex erection occurs as a result of external stimulation applied to the body below the level of the spinal cord lesion, generally to the pelvic organs. An effective stimulus may be touch applied to the external genitals or noxious stimuli such as pinching or pulling the pubic hair. Anal stimulation frequently causes erection in the male with complete spinal injury. Internal or visceral stimulation may be the cause of apparently spontaneous erections with stimuli originating most frequently from the bladder or rectum.

Reflex erections are seen most often in complete upper motor neuron lesions at any level but the maximal incidence is seen with lesions at the cervical level. This suggests that the longer is the intact and isolated spinal cord below the level of the injury the more likely is the autonomic reflex function of erection. This is also the case for the somatic reflex spasticity of skeletal muscles.

A few patients with complete upper motor neuron lesions may ejaculate. Their perception of this may be a strongly increased generalized spasticity before and extensor spasticity at the point where ejaculation would have occurred. This may be followed by complete flaccidity which may last for several hours. On the other hand, 20% of patients who have flaccid paraplegia due to a lower motor neuron lesion may ejaculate even though there is complete anesthesis of the skin and external genitals (Bors and Comarr, 1960).

The sensation of orgasm may or may not accompany the ejaculation. In the neurologically normal male, orgasm may occur in the absence of the seminal vesicles, vas deferens, or prostate. It can also occur in spite of denervation of the smooth muscles of the adnexa provided the muscles of the pelvic floor and skin of the genitals retain their innervation. In the paraplegic male, orgasm can occur in spite of denervation of the pelvic floor and genital skin if the smooth muscles or the adnexa retain their innervation. Ejaculation may be normal, or retrograde into the urinary bladder.

Some spinal injured males and females report orgasm in spite of complete denervation of all pelvic structures. Although this may be difficult for the able-bodied person to understand, it is reported to be entirely satisfying and leads to a comfortable resolution stage of sexual excitement. Indeed, some spinal injured adults state that they are able to concentrate on sensation from a neurologically intact portion of their bodies and reassign that sensation to their genitals, thus experiencing it in their fantasy as orgasm. Using that technique some spinal injured males report multiple orgasms.

The paraplegic or quadriplegic male who is unable to ejaculate is for all practical purposes infertile. However, there has been some experimentation with alternate methods of harvesting sperm. Intrathecal injections of Prostigmin have been used with variable success and have produced pregnancy in the spouse (Guttman and Walsh, 1971). Electrical stimulation of the seminal vesicles similar to that used in animal husbandry had also been tried, sometimes yielding significant counts of sperm (Bensman and Kottke, 1966). However, the sperm are characterized by abnormal forms, are relatively immotile, and thus ineffective for fertilization.

In recent years experimental work has been done with surgically implanted silicon prostheses to create or maintain the penis in the erect state. However, surgically implanted silicone prostheses as well as fluid transfer systems for the treatment of impotence are still experimental (Lash, 1968; Kotari et al., 1972).

Since many of the sexual responses of the human male are common knowledge, the spinal injured male can be directly compared to his able-bodied counterpart. What may be surprising to see in Table 4 is that the differences between the two are few and consist primarily of the paraplegic's and quadraplegic's difficulty in achieving emission and ejaculation. Penile erection is not as predictable nor caused by the same stimuli as for the ablebodied male, but the other features of the male sexual response cycle are more remarkable for their similarities than their differences. It may be of comfort to the recently injured male to learn that his sexual responsivity is not greatly different from what it was before. However, one must not minimize or deny the impact that the injury has had on his sexuality. Patients profit from having as much information as possible about their bodily responses and capabilities.

TABLE 4

Male sexual response cycle:
Comparison of sexual response cycles in able-bodied
and spinal cord injured males

	Able-Bodied Male	Spinal Cord Injured Male
Penis	Erects	Erects
Skin of scrotum	Tenses	Tenses
Testes	Elevate in scrotum	Elevate in scrotum
Emission	Yes	No
Ejaculation	Yes	No
Nipples	Erect	Erect
Muscles	Tense, spasms	Tense, spasms
Breathing rate	Increases	Increases
Pulse	Increases	Increases
Blood pressure	Increases	Increases
Skin of trunk, neck, face	Sex flush	Sex flush

FEMALE SEXUALITY AND SPINAL CORD INJURY

Approximately 80% of all spinal injured adults are males and most of the literature written on sexuality of spinal cord injury relates to the male. However, some information about the female is available. Most reports state that the female's sexuality is less devastated than the male's. This is not to deny the enormity of the injury upon the female but rather to point out differences in physiology, anatomy, and cultural expectation for the two sexes. Most people agree that in our culture it is probably easier for a female to adapt herself to a physically passive role in sexual activity than it is for a male. Thus the motor paralysis of spinal cord injury may be less threatening to her.

Certainly many women would strenuously disagree with the suggestion that females are more restricted in the physical activity or athletics of sex. However, the medical literature does stress this difference and emphasizes that women will generally find their sexual options less limited by motor and sensory paralysis than men. Certainly in terms of fertility, the female is virtually unaffected by spinal cord injury whereas the male's fertility is greatly reduced.

Changes in the menstrual patterns of women may occur as a result of spinal cord injury. Approximately 50% of women will be amenorrheic for a short period of time after the injury but almost all will experience a return of their normal menstrual cycle. Dysmenorrhea and dyspareunia, if present prior to injury, usually disappear with the loss of sensation resulting from the spinal cord injury. Orgasm is affected for women as it is for men. If the cord injury is complete there can be no appreciation of physical stimulation of the genitals. Through highly developed fantasy and erotic imagery, however, the female may develop the ability to experience the stages of arousal, plateau, orgasm, and resolution. As in the spinal cord injured male, neurologically intact body parts may become more highly eroticized than they were before paralysis.

Ovulation is unaffected by the injury and the female is capable of becoming pregnant and carrying a fetus to full term. Since the urinary tract is adversely affected by spinal cord injury and may also be by pregnancy, these two features are compounded. There is no indication that Cesarian section is any more indicated in paraplegic women than in able-bodied women. As one would expect, the uterus retains its ability to contract at the time of delivery but bearing down or voluntary assistance by the mother is necessarily limited. Premature labor is somewhat more of a hazard than in the neurologically intact woman. This is especially true if the spinal cord is injured above the 10th thoracic level. Labor pains may go unappreciated and the woman may find herself well along in labor before realizing it.

Episodic hypertension can be expected in that uncontrolled sympathetic overactivity is evoked in any spinal cord injured person whose injury is above the fourth thoracic segment. The obstetrician and anesthesiologist should be aware of the potential for autonomic hyperreflexia and its concomitant threat of severe systemic hypertension. However, the skilled medical team in an adequately equipped hospital should be able to manage this with little difficulty or risk.

Contraception may offer some special problems for the spinal cord injured female. Since there is an increased likelihood of pelvic and lower extremity venous thrombosis secondary to the spinal cord injury, the physician may be reluctant to prescribe oral contraceptive combinations of estrogen or progesterone because of their reported increase in thrombophlebitis. Similarly, the physician may be reluctant to recommend an intrauterine device in a patient whose sensory arc is damaged and who may not experience pelvic pain from migration of the device or incipient pelvic inflammatory disease.

Some physicians continue to believe that the woman in a wheelchair is unsuitable for raising small children and recommend that she avoid pregnancy. However, our experience has been that many women are capable of managing small children from their wheelchairs when they are provided with

TABLE 5

Female sexual response cycle:
Comparison of sexual response cycles in able-bodied
and spinal cord injured females

	Able-Bodied Female	Spinal Cord Injured Female
Wall of vagina	Moistens	
Clitoris	Swells	Swells
Labia	Swells and opens	Swells
Uterus	Contracts	
Inner 2/3 of vagina	Expands	
Outer 1/3 of vagina	Contracts	
Nipples	Erect	Erect
Muscles	Tense, spasms	Tense, spasms
Breasts	Swell	Swell
Breathing	Increases	Increases
Pulse	Increases	Increases
Blood pressure	Increases	Increases
Skin of trunk, neck, face	Sex flush	Sex flush

a reasonable amount of help consistent with their disability. This decision, of course, should be individualized and based upon the couple's wishes and their overall ability to adapt to the rehabilitation needs of the injured partner.

Just as for the male, the spinal cord injured female's sexual response cycle can be compared to that of her able-bodied counterpart (Table 5). Although less is known about the sexual responses of the paralyzed female than the male, some information is available. Again, the woman's sexual responses after spinal cord injury are more noted for their similarities than differences with respect to her neurologically intact sister.

A few key points in working with the spinal injured adult bear mentioning here. These apply almost equally to any sexually active adult who is in a position to reassess his attitudes, competence, and relationships. They are: ability to communicate effectively with one's partner, willingness to experiment with sexual options which are pleasing to both partners, use of pleasuring techniques, emphasis upon fantasy, the importance of hygiene, and recognition that the largest component of human sexual excitement and response remains undamaged within the skull. A satisfactory resolution of the sexual aspect of living may be of prime importance after spinal cord injury. This is true whether one elects sexual celibacy or indulgence. The choices should be made from a vantage point of information and as much freedom from ignorance and taboos as possible. The expectation that the patient is capable of a satisfying sexual life should be clear.

An especially difficult problem is created for the male with a flaccid penis which results from injury to the lower cord. Some men who are unable to achieve erections psychically or reflexly conclude that their sexual lives are over or limited. Therefore, for couples who consider intravaginal containment of the penis an important aspect of sexual activity, we teach the stuffing method, a technique which is a part of the sexual therapy sometimes utilized in the treatment of premature ejaculation. With cooperation and experimentation, a paralyzed male can be positioned above or below his female partner and his flaccid penis can be inserted or stuffed into her vagina. If the woman has trained herself to voluntarily control her pubococcygeus muscles she can contract around the penis and hold it within her vagina for the satisfaction of both partners. Some women report that they can create a tourniquet effect which causes the penis to become engorged and stiffened.

COUNSELING

Some physically disabled adults receive counseling which helps them to accommodate their sexual lives to their physical capacities, dispositions, and desires. However, most do not. The University of Minnesota has recently made attempts to bring counseling on a programmatic basis to each patient who wishes it. In order to facilitate this, a major segment of the clinical staff of the Rehabilitation Center participated in a Sexual Attitude Reassessment Seminar, the prototype of which was developed by the National Sex Forum, San Francisco, California (see Chapter 18). That model was modified for the specific needs of the professional staff of the Rehabilitation Center. The endorsement of this approach made it possible for human sexuality to take a respectable place with the other aspects of patient care in the Center. It soon became a staff expectation that the patient's sexuality would be dealt with openly in the same manner as was his locomotor, pulmonary, or gastrointestinal function. Patients eventually came to realize that sexual rehabilitation was a part of the treatment program and that they could ask questions of anyone on the Rehabilitation Team. Answers are provided wherever possible and if the staff member is unable to provide the requested information, he or she can obtain it from other members of the Team. This has made it possible for patients and their partners to utilize any relationship that has developed with a member of the hospital staff. The physician is not an essential person

TABLE 6

A REASONABLE HOSPITAL APPROACH	BECAUSE	BUT	AN ALTERNATE HOSPITAL APPROACH	BECAUSE
With regard to disabled patients, I'll leave the discussion of sex to someone who is effective.	I don't want to hurt the disabled.	Everyone else might do just as I do and the disabled will receive no help at all.	Try discussing sexuality with disabled patients.	Disabled people can 'take it.' They will appreciate your sensitivity and honest inquiry. The information will help them function in an able-bodied world.
With regard to my colleagues, I'll leave the discussion of sex to the specialists.	Sexuality is an intimate and private affair. Furthermore, I don't know enough about it to discuss it with my colleagues.	Others may not discuss it either and the topic may be overlooked entirely, leaving the patient uninformed and further disabled.	Talk with colleagues about natural human functions, including sexual function.	When sex is discussed a deliberate treatment plan can be formulated and a new disability may be avoided.
My primary responsibility is to help people achieve a better state of health. I'll work on that first.	Sex is separate from health and I'm too busy anyway. The patient will ask or take care of it himself if he really needs to know.	Perhaps no one will take responsibility for informing the disabled about their sexual potentials.	Initiate discussion, provide information and endorse sexuality with disabled patients.	Healthy sexuality is part of good mental health and we are responsible for helping people achieve a better state of health.
I will help people avoid the distractions of sex by concentrating their attention on their hospital care.	If I allow the distraction of sexuality, it may become unmanageable. It is not really that important to the hospital treatment anyway.	Sex as a natural part of life deserves encouragement and belongs in the hospitalization process.	Teach sexual awareness and responsibility as part of living.	Encourage sexual rehabilitation in the hospital as well as out of it. Learning should be expected just as people are expected to learn other new coping techniques of daily living.

Reality and responsibility, which are essential to learning, may be different for different people.	Human sexuality includes competence as well as relationships.	Sexuality is an early concern of many patients. Speaking about it directly will help set a rapport of honesty and responsibility.	To be helpful with another person's sexuality one must first be comfortable with his or her own.
Explain reality adequately to people. Then expect responsible action from them.	Give support and importance to the idea that sexual competence is also important. It helps us all feel good about ourselves.	Deal with personal aspects of hospitalization openly and sincerely.	Recognize that we are all sexual beings, endorse sexuality in terms of feelings.
My rules may not apply equally to all people.	By being so sure of myself I may make it difficult for patients to talk to me should their ideas be different from mine.	By denying that we all have sexual feelings we may inhibit their emergence in patients.	Some people are shy and lack permission to speak freely about sexuality.
People need rules for guidance.	My religion is a great help to me in understanding what is right and wrong in human sexuality.	The professional relationship insures objectivity. Besides, after injury physically disabled people don't have the same sexual feelings.	I will speak with propriety which will lend respect to the topic. It doesn't help the patient if he thinks I am "too free."
I expect people to abide by the same rules of responsibility and professionalism that I do.	Relationships and understanding are the essence of sexuality. When asked, I consider it my job to tell people what is right and wrong about sex.	No matter how personal they may sometimes seem, medical, nursing, and therapy procedures have to be done.	When appropriate, I answer the patient's questions about residual reproductive or sexual capacity.

in the counseling process although frequently is involved in that aspect of the counseling which involves medical or physiological considerations.

Where possible, partners are also involved in counseling. This is not always possible, since some people have no partners when they become disabled. Rather than deny them access to sexual counseling, it has been provided if desired. The nature of the counseling is quite different, however, since a person who has no partner with whom to share the counseling experience is greatly disadvantaged in dealing with attitudes and behaviors. Yet, many disabilities are characterized by precisely this absence of sexual partners. Requiring those counselees to participate as couples would be placing the cart before the horse.

In the hospital or health care facility it is unwise to wait for the patient to ask questions before providing information. Many patients are so overwhelmed by their disabilities that they will not ask questions. The professional should anticipate the need for counseling and provide it as appropriate. Some believe that it is inappropriate to provide counseling early in the hospital course. It has been our experience, however, that information is appreciated by most patients, some of whom simply store it for later use. In any event, the physician who is willing to discuss sexual aspects of a disability is likely to build a more secure rapport with the patient who now senses that the physician is indeed interested in him or her as a whole person and not only in damaged body portions.

There are some general guidelines for talking with the recently physically disabled patient in the hospital. Do not be frightened or put off by the patient. The disabled person can receive the information as well if not better than an able-bodied counterpart. Provide information in an understanding and sincere manner. Utilize eye contact to the extent that you can do so comfortably. Sanction sexuality as a normal and anticipated activity. Discuss sexuality in the context of the variety of problems which the patient faces. Do not make the subject conspicuous by segregating it for separate handling.

Rehabilitation begins as soon as the patient's life is no longer threatened and he or she has had a few days to think and contemplate the post-hospital adjustment. This is an appropriate time to begin frank discussion of losses caused by the disability. Discussion should include physical, occupational, personal, and recreational loss. The patient's ability to perform or achieve should also be discussed frankly. He should be encouraged to remember those things done in the past and begin to anticipate those that are possible in the future. The ability to perform can easily be related to sexuality. Can he masturbate? Does he think he will be fertile? Does he consider himself as an acceptable marriage partner? It is appropriate at this time to talk about the patient's partner. Perhaps he or she has questions which can assist the patient in beginning to deal with this aspect of hospitalization.

Table 6 summarizes some of the ways in which hospital staffs have dealt with their patients in various aspects of sexuality. It is neither inclusive nor typical but is rather a grouping of a variety of common situations. The first column of Table 6 lists some hospital staff behaviors or approaches. The second column suggests why that approach is employed. The third column points out some undesirable side effects which are based upon the approach and rationale in the first two columns. The fourth and fifth columns, respectively, suggest an alternate approach for dealing with a patient's sexuality in the hospital and a rationale upon which that alternate approach is based.

There are many old and contradictory myths about sex and physical disability. Together with a lack of information and feelings of guilt about the sexual capabilities of disabled people, they produce an avoidance of honest and helpful exchange between patient and doctor. Almost all physically disabled adults can expect to enjoy an active sex life.

REFERENCES

Bennedick, T. G. 1971. Disease as Aphrodisiac. Bull. Hist. Med. 45: 433-340.
Bensman, A. and Kottke, F. J. 1966. Induced Emission of Sperm Utilizing Electrical Stimulation of the Seminal Vesicles and Vas Deferens. Arch. Phys. Med. 47: 436-443.
Bors, E. and Comarr, A. E. 1960. Neurological Disturbances of Sexual Function with Special Reference to 529 Patients with Spinal Cord Injury. Urol. Surv. 10: 191-222.
Cole, T. M., Chilgren, R., and Rosenberg, P. 1973. A new Programme of Sex Education and Counseling for Spinal Cord Injured Adults and Health Care Professionals. Int. J. Paraplegia. 11: 111-124.
Comarr, A. E. 1970. Sexual Function among Patients with Spinal Cord Injury. Urol. Int. 25: 134-168.
Easton, J. K. M. Excerpted 1973 from an unpublished essay.
Ehrlich, G.E. (Ed.): Total Management of the Arthritic Patient. pp. 193–208. Philadelphia: J. B. Lippincott Co.
Finley, F. R. 1972. Research and Training Accomplishments in Bioengineering. Conference in Rehabilitation Research and Training Center. Philadelphia.
Fox, J. 1971. Sex Education—but for What? Spec. Educ. 60: 15-17.
Guttman, L. and Walsh, J. J. 1971. Prostigmin Assessment of Fertility in Spinal Man. *Paraplegia* 9: 39-51.
Herman, M. 1950. Role of Somesthetic Stimuli in the Development of Sexual Excitation in Man. Arch. Neurol. Psychiat. 64: 42-56.
Jocheim, K. A. and Wahle, H. 1970. A Study on Sexual Function in 56 Male Patients with Complete Irreversible Injuries of the Spinal Cord and Cauda Equina. Paraplegia 8: 166-169.
Kotari, D. R., Timm, G. W., Frohrib, D. A., and Bradley, W. E. 1972. An Implantable Fluid Transfer System for Treatment of Impotence. J. Biometrics 5: 567-570.
Krusen, F. H., Kottke, F. J., and Ellwood, P. M., Jr. (eds.) 1973. *Handbook of Physical Medicine and Rehabilitation.* (2nd Ed.) Philadelphia: W. B. Saunders. pp. 193-208.

Lash, H. 1968. Silicone Implant for Impotence. J. Urol. 100: 709-710.

Linder, H. 1953. Perceptual Sensitization to Sexual Phenomena in the Chronic Physically Handicapped. J. Clin. Psychol. 9: 67-68.

Money, J. 1967. In (C. W. Wahl, ed.). pp. 226-287. *Sexual Problems: Diagnosis and Treatment in Medical Practice.* New York: Free Press.

Mooney, T. O., Cole, T. M., and Chilgren, R. A. Sexual Options for Paraplegia and Quadriplegia. To be published.

Richardson, S. A. 1972. People with Cerebral Palsy Talk for Themselves. Dev. Med. Child Neurol. 14: 524-535.

Tsuji, I., Nakajima, F., Morimoto, J., and Nounaka, Y. 1961. The Sexual Function in Patients with Spinal Cord Injury. Urol. Int. 12: 270-280.

Weiss, A. J. and Diamond, M. 1966. Sexual Adjustment, Identification, and Attitudes of Patients with Myelopathy. Arch. Phys. Med. 47: 245-250.

Zeitlin, A. B., Cottrell, T. L., and Lloyd, F. A. 1957. Sexology of the Paraplegic Male. J. Fertil. Steril. 8: 377-344.

chapter

13

Threat of heart attack for the middle-age male carries ominous overtones—instant death, survival with semi-invalid status, and fear of recurrence upon physical exertion. Termination of sexuality is frequently considered a consequence of myocardial infarction. The fear of sudden death during intercourse hovers as a personal cloud which halts the sexual relationship of many couples. Is termination necessary? Does energy expenditure during intercourse significantly endanger the cardiac patient? What are the research facts? Practical guidelines for the post-heart-attack patient can be rationally developed and presented.

Editor

172

Sexual Activity
and the Cardiac Patient

NATHANIEL N. WAGNER, Ph.D.

The World Health Organization has stated that ischemic heart disease has reached enormous proportions, striking more and more at younger people. Over 14,000,000 Americans of all ages and socioeconomic levels are afflicted with some form of heart or blood vessel ailment. Despite these large numbers, specific guidelines regarding the sexual adjustment of cardiac patients are scarce in the extensive literature on cardiovascular disease. Little is empirically established about the effects of particular forms of sexual activity upon the diseased or damaged heart and the cardiovascular system in general.

An example of medical difficulty in dealing with sexuality can be seen in an otherwise excellent epidemiological and prospective study of coronary heart disease. Morris *et al* (1973) have described their questionnaire study in which subjects were asked to "record everything they would normally discuss with another person, which... imposes limitations." No definition of what one "would normally discuss with another person" was given. Not surprisingly, there is not a single mention of sexual activity in this study although there are detailed data on swimming, tennis, sailing as crew, hill climbing, dancing, morning exercises, gardening, brisk walking, running, cycling, and climbing stairs.

Standard recommendations to the coronary patient typically include reducing or stopping smoking, weight reduction, cholesterol intake reduction, and regular physical exercise of a mild nature. Not much about sexual matters. Consequently the patient acts according to his limited knowledge, fears, opinions, or superstitions. He may make unwarranted reductions in sexual activity, even to the point of abstinence. This begins a cycle of behavior that may hamper full rehabilitation. The reduced sexual activity can lead to frustration and marital conflicts, factors guaranteed to impede recovery and often associated with an increase in cardiac symptomatology.

In order to forestall this cycle, the physician should be direct and specific in advising cardiac patients about their sexual activity. The physician must have good information about the impact of sexual activity on the damaged heart.

PHYSIOLOGY OF INTERCOURSE

The physiological effects of sexual intercourse have been studied only in recent years. These studies, however, have been conducted in artificial laboratory settings with healthy young subjects. The data obtained from such studies (Masters and Johnson, 1966) suggest that sexual activity is associated with marked cardiovascular fluctuations including tachycardia ranging from 110 to 180 beats per min. and impressive increases in blood pressure, 40 to 80 mm. systolic and 20 to 50 mm. diastolic. Respiratory rates also increase to 30 to 60 per min.

Although these changes are dramatic, they are also quite brief, with a gradual build-up in blood pressure, respiratory rate, and heart rate to a peak just before, or simultaneous with orgasm, and followed by a drop to normal levels over the next few minutes.

But what is the impact of sexual activity on the man with a diseased cardiovascular system? A recent study by Hellerstein and Friedman (1970) reports the first significant effects of sexual activity and other daily activity in arteriosclerotic heart-diseased patients, and in normal coronary-prone patients. It also examines the relationships between various social and psychological factors, and sexual activity. The investigators concluded that for the middle-aged, middle-class, long-married man, the physiological cost of sexual activity is modest, especially when compared to the physiological impact of sexual activity upon young volunteers in laboratory settings. Heart rate response with the older patients was minimal, with peak heart rate averaging 117.4 per min. (range 90 to 140). Heart rates for min. 2 and 1 before the peak heart rate were 87 and 101, and 96 and 85, 1 and 2 min. after peak rate.

Responses are similar to those observed in the same individuals during regular daily activity, such as driving a car, discussing business matters or climbing one or two flights of stairs. Blood pressure was not measured during sexual activity, but was measured in these patients during bicycle exercise testing, providing a comparison between heart rate and blood pressure response to exercise.

If these two forms of exercise are considered equivalent, it can be predicted that the average blood pressure at rest before sexual activity was 127/85 and rose to 162/89 at peak heart rate during sexual intercourse. There are several reasons, however, to doubt that the blood pressure and heart rate responses are similar in these two forms of physical exercise.

It is known that exercise, such as running on a treadmill or bicycle exercise, while elevating the cuff blood pressure in the arms, does not actually elevate central aortic blood pressure. Isometric contraction of even small muscle groups, such as sustained hand grip, has a profound hypertensive effect on both cuff and central aortic blood pressure. It seems possible that sexual intercourse performed in the male-on-top position results in sustained isometric arm and shoulder contraction. If this is so, it is therefore likely that blood pressure changes during intercourse performed in some positions may be elevated out of proportion to the modest elevations in heart rate reported by Hellerstein and Friedman. It is well known that central aortic blood pressure or left ventricular afterload is an important determinant of myocardial oxygen consumption. Marked increases in afterload have the potential of precipitating angina, myocardial infarction, and serious or fatal arrhythmias. Because of the detrimental effect of isometric exercise, coronary patients are cautioned against activity such as lifting heavy objects, carrying suitcases and snow shoveling, which involve this type of muscular work. In addition, we believe that male patients should be advised to initially perform sexual intercourse in positions such that they will not have to support their body with their arms for sustained periods. Side-by-side and female-on-top are two positions which are desirable for the male from this point of view. For females, male superior, female superior and side-by-side positions would not present isometric arm or shoulder muscle contraction. Therefore, the issue of coital position is less important for females.

THE COITAL CORONARY

A common concern among patients, their spouses, and their physicians is the danger of a coital coronary. Although they admit that sexual activity *can* result in acute coronary insufficiency and death among cardiac patients, Hellerstein and Friedman maintain that probably only a small percentage of deaths among cardiac patients is attributable to sexual activity. Those deaths that do occur do not involve the middle-aged, middle-class males who engage in sexual activity with their wives of 20 years or more, and who are statistically more coronary prone. There is suggestive evidence, however, that nonmarital sexual activities undertaken by married males may lead to much more profound physiological changes, including severe elevation in both heart rate and blood pressure. There is good reason to believe that such sexual activity with new or newer partners is particularly stress-producing. It appears likely that most episodes of sudden death during sexual intercourse occur under these conditions. Obviously, therefore, such activity should be avoided, although counseling the patient in this area requires considerable tact.

It is important to note that it is the newness and unfamiliarity of the partner that increases the risk. Similarly, a man resuming sexual activity with his wife after a 10-year period of abstinence would be at great risk. The principle is that any new anxiety-arousing activity will cause increases in a wide variety of physiological parameters, including heart rate and blood pressure. The married or nonmarried aspect is only related to the newness and anxiety arousing dimensions.

MASTURBATION

Masturbation in relation to the cardiac patient has been unavailable for open discussion until very recently. It is extraordinarily important, however. The average patient with a myocardial infarct feels a severe threat to his sexual life. It has been demonstrated that there is a considerable development of impotency, most probably of psychogenic origin, following myocardial infarction. In one report (Tuttle *et al.* 1964) approximately 10% of the patients studied were no longer sexually functional.

When the male patient is out of the acute phase of illness, when cardiac monitoring is no longer indicated, and when the individual begins to walk about the hospital, it is not uncommon for sexual concern and interest to develop. A number of male patients have reported that female nurses at this point become more sexually attractive each day.

For many male patients the return of sexual arousal is a welcome sign of rehabilitation and the potential for a normal life. Interviews with patients indicate that it is not uncommon for the cardiac patient to masturbate while still in the hospital. This masturbation can be seen as an extraordinarily positive event from the point of view of a continuing sexual life. One individual indicated that he was relieved and joyous at being able to develop an erection and masturbate to orgasm although he was flooded with guilt at the same time. Despite the obvious advantage of masturbation over coitus for the resumption of sexual activity in cardiac patients, this matter has been neither studied nor discussed. Masters and Johnson (1966) in their exhaustive study of human sexual response, while detailing very clearly the cardiac cost of coitus, provide no explicit data on the cardiac cost of masturbation. In addition to the possibility of a lessened cardiac cost, there is the lessened problem of the interpersonal interaction when a male resumes sex relations with his former partner. The anxiety that she may feel about his condition and his performance exacerbates his anxiety and fears.

In a study presently being carried out at the University of Washington School of Medicine, we are measuring the cardiac cost of masturbation. Starting initially with healthy young males, we intend to also measure healthy young females and, later, cardiac patients. In our preliminary data on young males, it is clear that at the time of orgasm by masturbation the heart rate does not go above 130 and it rises to the 110 to 130 level for the briefest moments. These preliminary data are on 10 males, three trials each. This is in contrast to a cardiac cost of up to 180 for coital activity of individuals in this same health and age classification.

Physicians should consider discussing the therapeutic use of masturbation as a method of re-entrance into sexual activity for cardiac patients. Obviously, the physician needs to be sensitive to the patient's emotional and religious belief systems so as not to be crude or offensive. Nonetheless, the suggestion could be made to all patients that if they do not find the concept wrong from an ethical or moral point of view there is no contraindication to their masturbating as a way of renewing sexual activity. The physician can make this recommendation at a point in which he feels the patient has recovered sufficiently to where an accelerated heart rate of 130 beats per min. is not contraindicated.

COUNSELING THE PATIENT

Interaction among various physiological factors makes the problem of counseling the coronary patient especially difficult. When and to what extent can he resume sexual activity? The physician should take several factors into account: the general health of the patient; the extent of recovery from the coronary episode; physical activity level of the patient; fatiguability; the physiological cost of sexual activity; the emotional characteristics of the patient; and, most important, the extent of his precoronary sexual activity. Such knowledge is helpful but is not available in all instances. In terms of the resumption of sexual activity, however, minimum considerations should be the extent of recovery, the physiological costs of sexual activity, and the level of precoronary sexual activity. The last point is important because of the great variation in what can be termed "normal" sexual activity levels. What is comfortable for a given individual is what should be considered normal, and indeed optimal.Thus, the therapeutic goal would be a return to premorbid levels of sexual activity. We should not impose on the sexually nonactive patient the additional task of resuming sexual activity which may have been dormant for years.

Another salient factor is the role of the patient's spouse. Typically she is fearful and anxious about her husband's welfare. She sometimes becomes overprotective, often attempting to reduce her husband's responsibilities and activities, including sexual ones. He, in turn, may feel like an invalid, worthless, ineffectual, and potentially impotent. Such difficulties can be alleviated by counseling the spouse as well as the patient. Her expectations can then be realistic, her fears allayed, and her role delineated. Knowing that the physiological cost of sexual activity is minimal, and being aware of further means of reducing these costs, *e.g.,* side-by-side or female-on-top intercourse, makes the spouse a valuable asset during the recovery period.

The research cited and our own comments are concerned primarily with the male coronary patient. The preponderance of cardiac disease among males is well known. Females, however, do have cardiac problems. While studies of the relationships between sexual activity and the diseased heart among males are scarce, we have been unable to find *any* published studies or comments in textbooks on cardiology concerning the sexual activity of females.

The question remains, when should the patient be advised to resume sexual activity, following a myocardial infarction? Based on the above physiological research, when the patient has recovered to the point where he is able to climb one or two flights of stairs or walk several blocks at a brisk pace, the resumption of sexual intercourse should present no special hazard. If the patient experiences angina with brisk walking or stair climbing, prophylactic nitroglycerin may be useful to prevent angina during intercourse. Patients with congestive heart failure or general debilitation should be advised not to undertake strenuous physical activity, including sexual activity, until heart failure is controlled and general rehabilitation achieved.

When the patient has returned to mild to moderate physical activity, he can also return to the level of sexual activity he was experiencing prior to the onset of cardiac difficulties. Patients should not be deprived of assistance in this area of their rehabilitation.

REFERENCES

Hellerstein, H. K. and Friedman, E. H. 1970. Sexual Activity and the Post-Coronary Patient. Arch. Intern. Med., 125: 987-999.

Massie, E., Rose, E., Rupp, J., and Whelton, R. 1969. Sudden Death during Coitus—fact or fiction? Med. Aspects Human Sexuality. June, p. 22.

Masters, W. and Johnson, V. 1966. *Human Sexual Response.* Boston: Little, Brown.

Morris, J. N., Chave, S. P. W., Adam, C., Sirey, C., Epstein, L., and Sheehan, D. J. 1973. Vigorous Exercise in Leisure-Time and the Incidence of Coronary Heart Disease. Lancet, 17 February, 333-339.

Scheingold, L. D. and Wagner, N. N. 1974. *Sound Sex and the Aging Heart.* New York: Human Sciences Press.

Trimble, G. S. 1970. The Coital Coronary. Med Aspects Human Sexuality. May, 64-72.

Tuttle, W. B., Cook, W. L. Jr., and Fitch, E. 1964. Sexual Behavior in Post-Myocardial Infarction Patients. Am. J. Cardiol. 13: 140.

Veno, M. 1969. The So-Called Coital Death. Jap. J. Legal Med. 17: 535

chapter

14

Three percent of the population is mentally retarded. Do the mentally retarded have similar sexual interests as the nonretarded? Can they function effectively for pregnancy prevention when they wish it, and parenting when they wish that? Should they be rendered infertile? If the retarded individual has a child, will the child be similarly deficient in intellectual functioning?

These questions preoccupy the parents of the retarded, and are especially salient to the retarded patient. The physician must be able to assist. But, first, an understanding of the sexual functioning of the retarded as well as their capacity for pregnancy prevention and effective parenting is imperative. With this information, clinicians can sensibly counsel these millions of patients and their families.

Editor

Sexuality and the Mentally Retarded

JUDY E. HALL, Ph.D.

Expression of sexuality by those defined as mentally retarded has been historically (and is sometimes presently) handled by repressive techniques such as segregation from society and demands for sterilization. This has been accompanied by the creation of stereotypes and myths surrounding that expression. In looking at the advances made in the field of mental retardation—those relating to etiology, treatment of specific behavior and learning difficulties, or successful intervention with socioeconomic groups at high risk for incurring retardation—we have come to recognize the relative stagnation in another area. This is the sociosexual domain. It is now time to examine the sexuality of these members of society with a view toward enabling them to achieve enjoyment in life to the fullest extent of their capabilities.

Definition of Mental Retardation

In the United States the definition used to identify the mentally retarded is the one used by the American Association on Mental Deficiency: "Mental retardation refers to significantly subaverage general intellectual functioning, existing concurrently with deficits in adaptive behavior, and manifested during the developmental period." Although this definition stresses that adaptive behaviors must be deficited along with subaverage intellectual functioning, in actual practice individuals whose intelligence measures below an IQ of 70 are classified as mentally retarded on the basis of psychometric testing alone. Since adaptive behavior refers to the effectiveness with which

181

the individual meets the standards of personal independence and social responsibility expected of his age and cultural group, we are looking more at adaptive behavior than at intellectual behaviors when we examine sexuality. Presumably these adaptive behaviors are more readily changed while, in contrast, intellectual ability is seen as relatively immune to change. In addition, one must be careful not to assume that, because a person has a low measured intelligence, adaptive behaviors are similarly evaluated. In relation to sexuality, in fact, only rarely does the sexual development and expression of the retarded differ significantly from that of the "normal" population—although exceptional in certain areas, the mentally retarded are not exceptional in sexual impulses (Gordon and Green, 1972).

Two Major Categories of the Mentally Retarded

For the purpose of describing sexual expression, the population of the retarded will be divided into two groups. Group I is characterized by organic pathology of the central nervous system. Group I mental retardation can generally occur in all socioeconomic, ethnic, and racial groups. Since this first group is usually associated with measured intelligence of less than 55, these persons function at the trainable level or below in formal school settings (not expected to achieve functionally useful academic skills, so that self-care and social adjustment are envisioned as the goals of their schooling). Concomitant with this moderate to profound mental retardation are associated secondary physical disabilities. This group constitutes approximately 10 to 20% of the total population of the mentally retarded (the population of the mentally retarded is estimated at 3% of the total population of the United States). The etiology is any one of the hundreds of specific diseases and conditions which have been known to produce damage to the brain and to eventuate in retardation. People characterized as Group I are most frequently found in institutions or in direct supervision situations, and most are unlikely to move out into the community (Heber, 1970).

Group II constitutes the remaining 80 to 90% of the mentally retarded, and does not always present obvious or demonstrable gross pathology of the central nervous system. This group is characterized by mild intellectual deficit, resulting in an IQ range from 55 to 70 and a functioning in school at the educable level (can achieve academic work at least to the third grade level and occasionally to the sixth grade by school-leaving age). In adaptive behavior group II usually exhibits moderate or mild impairment. Although the basic cause of this type of retardation is unknown, evidence suggests possible inherited determinants, frequently in combination with conditions correlated with low socioeconomic status (high rates of prematurity, inadequate infant health supervision, lack of sufficient social interaction). Within the general population there is a particular segment which seems responsible for a high proportion of this type of retardation, often called cultural-familial retardation (Heber, 1970). An early diagnosis in group II retardation is not always stable, and the label of mental retardation may be confined only to a period in the child's daily life equivalent to 6 hr. a day—those hours alloted to learning experiences in the school situation. Very often, once they are adults, these "retarded" persons become less obviously deficient as members of society and no longer function as incompetently as they did while under the stress of school (President's committee, 1969).

Parents' Typical Reactions to Sexual Expression in Their Retarded Adolescent

In trying to understand the parents' point of view with regard to the expression of sexuality in the retarded, one further generalization might be helpful: the discrepancy between the IQ of the retarded adolescent and the IQ's (averaged) of the parents may predict, to a degree, how accepting those parents are of a retarded child. Extrapolating further, it predicts how the parents may react to sexual expression in that adolescent (Tarjan, 1971). If the parents' IQ average is close to that of their retarded adolescents (such as might be expected in cultural-familial retardation) sexual expression in that retarded person predictably would be accepted by the parents and seen as more similar to their own sexuality. Sexual expression in these cases is less devastating and less anxiety-provoking to the parents than it would be to those parents whose IQ's may be significantly discrepant from their adolescent. In this latter case, all the adolescent's social situations are extremely threatening to the parents. As a result, willful ignorance of the emergence of sexuality, and even suppression of sexual expression, may follow.

In addition to this parent *vs* child IQ discrepancy overview, there are more specific types of responses to sexuality that may arise from parents. From one pole—that of the secure, relatively well-adjusted parent—one often hears something like: "My child is as entitled as anyone to a natural sex life. He has the same needs for physical release and emotional closeness. If he meets someone he can go on loving, and who returns love, they should marry and be given whatever support is necessary to make the marriage work. The question of children requires serious thought and planning". (Goodman, 1972).

At the opposite pole, there are a variety of responses from families who are less well-adjusted regarding sexuality (Goodman):

1. *Denial of Sexuality.* The parent views the adolescent as a child, without strong physical urges, and denies that the adolescent often thinks about sex. Often the parent feels that to talk about sex might stir up ideas that aren't there, and thinks that it's better that the adolescent be kept innocent.

2. *Pseudo-Enlightened Attitude.* The parent agrees only to a narrow definition of sexuality, or restricts the adolescent sufficiently so that there is little opportunity for sociosexual interaction.

3. *Vicarious Sexuality.* The parent unconsciously encourages the acting out of his or her own sexual fantasies, while holding the retarded child later accountable for this unacceptable behavior. (This may be signified by excessive concern on the parent's part over minor dangers and enticements (Johnson and Szurek, 1952).)

4. *Moralistic Attitude: "Sex is Sinful."* This response envisions sex as permissible only in marriage and primarily for the purpose of procreation. This response is one of the most difficult to deal with, since simultaneously with this attitude comes the belief that the retarded person is incapable of accepting marital responsibilities. Therefore, any expression of sexuality is viewed with alarm.

5. *Over-Protective Attitude: "Sex is Too Risky."* This last approach is one that "endangers the retarded person's human dignity and tends to keep him from experiencing the normal taking of risks in life which is necessary for human growth and development" (Perske, 1972). The retarded person is over-protected and emotionally smothered, and therefore sexual expression is seen as too risky to engage in.

Fortunately, the most frequent response encountered is the honest, searching one of "I don't know; I want to do the right thing, but I don't know what is appropriate."

Interaction with Parents of the Retarded

It is essential that the person dealing with the sexual behavior of the retarded be as nonjudgmental as possible. In some families one can talk openly about sexual matters and in others there is a taboo. It is helpful, then, to respect the family's attitudes when dealing with the mentally retarded. Some attitudes of parents toward the retarded regarding sexual rights and expressions of sexuality reflect, at the least, ambivalence. Personal family dynamics become involved due to unresolved conflicts over the members' own sexuality, lack of knowledge and sophistication about sexual matters, and discomfort at discussing the subject with others. Frequently many parents are also bound by social or religious values about sexual behavior. In addition, they may worry about the possibility of their child producing another retarded child. Even though many parents are interested in participating in sex education programs, approaching them through factual discussions and/or professional encouragement may not be enough since their view of their child's sexuality is intermeshed into their whole pattern of reaction to having a retarded child. These responses of parents are often brought about only in adolescence, with the emergence of sexuality to the point where it can no longer be ignored. By that time it may be too late to develop in the retarded an attitude toward healthy sexual expression or in the parent a tolerance toward that expression.

PROBLEMS AND ALTERNATIVE SOLUTIONS

In attempting to address the concerns of parents and of the general population, some of the history and the relatively limited literature available on the sexual development and sexual expression of the retarded will be summarized. Additionally, specific recommendations will be made where appropriate.

Sexual Development, Masturbation, Exploitation, Homosexuality, and Venereal Disease

The sexuality of the retarded has been an area in which there have been frequent and often contradictory myths. Examples are: "The mentally retarded are oversexed"; "Severely and profoundly retarded adolescents are infertile"; "Frequent masturbation by the mentally retarded adolescent will lead to physical or mental harm"; "Retarded persons stay children forever"; "All mentally retarded children are late in maturing sexually"; "Mentally retarded persons are undersexed" (Hall, 1974). As would be expected, there are no simple explanations for the falsity of these statements. However, the simplest rule to follow is that, with few exceptions, the sexual development and expression of the retarded corresponds to the pattern found in the "normal" population.

The best studies evaluating sexual maturation in the mentally retarded show a delay in sexual development as IQ decreases (Flory, 1936; Mosier *et al.* 1962). However, the various syndromes of mental retardation (except for Down's syndrome) do not seem to account for the dissimilar patterns of growth between individuals. (As is true with most of the characteristics of the mentally retarded, there is variability in their sexual developmental indices also.) Sexual expression by group II mentally retarded persons is likely to be initially auto-erotic and later hetero- or homosexual. Group I is likely to engage only in self-stimulating behavior, although those with IQ's in the 40 to 55 range may develop attachments much like those of Group II. In general, then, it can be said that the sexual development pattern of the retarded follows the usual pattern, though with some lag in time.

Masturbation concerns most parents, and especially parents who have mentally retarded adolescents. Behavior which is acceptable when practiced by a normal person sometimes becomes unacceptable when practiced by someone who is different. Although some training may be necessary as to the place where masturbation is permitted, what needs to be stressed to parents is that masturbation is a normal phenomenon, not conducive to harm, and capable of giving a great deal of satisfaction. What needs to be taught is the following:

1. Masturbation is a normal expression of sex, no matter how frequently it is done or at what age. It becomes a compulsive, punitive, self-destructive behavior largely as a result of guilt, suppression, and punishment.

2. All direct sexual behavior involving the genitals should be in privacy. Recognizing that institutions for the retarded are not built or developed to insure privacy, the definition of what constitutes privacy in an institution must be very liberal. Bathrooms, one's own bed, the bushes, and the basement are private domain (Gordon and Green, 1972).

Should masturbatory behavior occur in inappropriate places, the mentally retarded have to be made to realize that this is private place behavior. The adolescent should be asked to go where there is privacy. No punishment should be administered. With consistency, firmness, and repetition, this response will be learned, much as toilet training was acquired. The administration of tranquilizers is to be avoided, since this generally is ineffective where masturbation is concerned and may affect other behaviors adversely in the form of a very pronounced general retardation.

Another frequent concern of parents of the retarded is the fear that their adolescent, usually a female, will be exploited sexually. Often this fear is presented in the context of a request for sterilization. Sometimes the subtle assumption is made by the parent that if one sterilizes then one destroys not only the ability to procreate but total sexuality as well. Or, this fear of sexual exploitation may relate to an even greater fear that, should exploitation occur and conception take place, the parent would have the responsibility for another retarded child. Besides recommending temporary methods of contraception instead of sterilization, it is also recommended that the parents be counseled that their handling of any sexual exploitation episode determines how traumatic that experience may be for the adolescent. Verbal admonishment concerning how to avoid this type of situation will not be enough for the mentally retarded; in sex education classes it can be helpful if these types of situations are role-played, so that specific behaviors can be learned. For example, the teacher can play the person who invites the retarded adolescent to get into a car (as the Kinsey female sample shows, this frequently may be someone known to the family rather than the proverbial stranger). Alternate ways to handle the situation could then be enacted by members of the class.

Homosexual relationships of the retarded, as with the normal IQ person, are likely to occur especially where heterosexual expression is not allowed (Gordon and Green, 1972). A retarded person might also choose an individual of the same sex for a focus in socio-sexual expression. Although society presently frowns on homosexuality as a mode of sexual expression, attitudes are changing with regard to what is viewed as "abnormal" or "deviant." The possibility of this orientation being an alternate model for the retarded cannot be dismissed without due consideration.

An additional concern is the possibility of venereal disease. It is reported that the incidence in the retarded population is three times the rate in the normal IQ population (Kempton, 1973). Although periodic checkups can include tests for syphilis and gonorrhea, parents and the mentally retarded should be educated as to the symptoms.

Contraception

There is no formal research evaluating the methods of contraception available when used with the mentally retarded (except for sterilization). However, recommendations have been made as to the method of choice for certain groups (Fujita *et al*, 1970; LaVeck and de la Cruz, 1973). Combining these recommendations with the parent-adolescent IQ discrepancy formulation, it is possible to generate some tentative guesses as to which methods would be acceptable and, perhaps, most effective. If the parents' IQ is only slightly higher than that of a group II individual, as is typical of cultural-familial retardation, it is unlikely that the parent will see a need for birth control. Those characterized as group I could benefit from birth control, but if the parents' IQ average is considerably higher than that of their adolescent, this family is going to be most insistent on sterilization. Equipped with information regarding the possible side-effects of the methods of contraception, the approach to these two family situations would be the same: the encouragement of temporary methods of contraception, such as the intrauterine device for group I, and either the IUD or oral contraceptives for group II. Oral contraceptives are most appropriate for mildly retarded women who function under high motivation and regular supervision; the IUD is best for sexually active women who lack motivation and supervision. Unfortunately, with the exception of vasectomy, the responsibility for controlling conception at the present time must rest on the female retarded. The condom is likely to be too difficult a procedure to be of any use to either group II or group I males. Although there are prospective methods of contraception that might be useful with the retarded population, most of the other methods now available are seen as too difficult for the retarded to learn. (If conception takes place, two alternatives available today for use with the mentally retarded are abortion and amniocentesis [to help rule out certain forms of genetic retardation] where appropriate.) In view of the alternative methods available and in view of the lack of information demonstrating whether the retarded person can use temporary contraceptive methods, many feel it is irrational to recommend sterilization as the only means of reproductive control (Fujita *et al.*, 1970).

Sterilization

Beginning in the early 1900's, at the peak of the eugenics movement when all mental retardation was thought hereditary and people were concerned with preventing the "unfit" from procreating, sterilizations were frequently performed on those housed in institutions. At this time, the "unfit" not only included those defined (rather loosely) as mentally retarded, but also the mentally ill, the epileptic, and the socially deviant (Butler, 1945). However, by the middle 1940's, the enthusiasm for this permanent method of birth control had diminished for primarily two reasons: 1) the discovery that only a small proportion of mental retardation was due to genetic causes, and

2) recognition of the low reproductive rate of the mentally retarded (Hall, 1974). Not surprisingly, at no time during the wholesale sterilization of the retarded was there interest evinced in the retarded's personal viewpoint on sterilization. However, several years later, a group of the mentally retarded was interviewed—50 individuals who had been released from the institution on the condition that each be sterilized (Edgerton, 1967). Although this interviewing was done many years after the operation, most had a vivid recollection of the procedure and saw sterilization as a permanent brand, reminding them of the humiliation of being labeled mentally retarded and of being placed in an institution.

Legal Aspects of Mandated and Voluntary Sterilization

With the abandonment of compulsory sterilization—though not with the repeal of any of the state statutes regarding sterilization—voluntary sterilization was suggested as an alternative procedure. But here a problem arose that is still with us—that of obtaining a truly informed consent from the mentally retarded. The same behavioral characteristics which suggest the necessity for permanent birth control probably obviate the possibility of informed consent. The inherent difficulty in obtaining true consent is best stated as follows (Tarjan, 1971):

1. Since the mentally retarded are not sufficiently competent to authorize surgical procedures and since they are highly suggestible and easily influenced by authoritative figures, *their* consent cannot be considered as truly informed;

2. *Parents* are too emotionally involved with the topic of sexuality in their adolescents to reach an objective decision on sterilization; and

3. *Arbitors* and/or *guardians* may not be able to rationally decide what is at best, based on symptomatology present today in the adolescent but which might not be present at a later date.

With current methods for preventing pregnancy, sterilization presents problems of obtaining informed consent, and because of the present irreversibility of the procedures is an unnecessarily restrictive alternative. It is hoped that the decision to sterilize will no longer be made perfunctorily. It is also reported that some mentally retarded adults who have requested the operation have sometimes been unable to obtain it (M. Bass, personal communication, 1973). Therefore, it is hoped that the procedure will still be made available to those who desire it and to those who are in a position to make the decision carefully, but with all other alternatives examined.

Marriage

Marriage for the mentally retarded has historically been linked to reproduction; hence the enactment of statutes preventing marriage in many of the states. Now that procreation is no longer a given in marriage, and now that birth control devices are available which more nearly control procreation, we need to re-examine the possible gains obtained from a marital relationship, as well as the risks. It is likely that a majority of group II retarded will marry, whereas a minority of group I will marry. In the past more retarded females than males have married. Most studies which have evaluated marriage in the mentally retarded have done so in the context of evaluating other variables conducive to community placement. Therefore, the subjects of these studies had once been institutionalized. The evaluation usually was in the form of a rating of the "goodness" of the marriage, or a determination of the divorce rate (Hall, 1974). More recent and better studies have individually interviewed each couple. In one study, the marriage pattern was not noticeably different from that of persons with similar socioeconomic status; in fact, the marital and sexual lives were more "normal" than would have been predicted on the basis of IQ and the behaviors which led to institutionalization (Edgerton, 1967). In the other study, in which both members of the couple were retarded, approximately 60% of the couples were rated as having a supportive and affectionate relationship. These marriages worked on a complementary basis—the skill of one person supplementing the inability of the other. Many marriages were "cocooned" and did not rely on outside help (Mattinson, 1973).

Affectional needs met in a close interpersonal relationship, even for a short period of time and at some expense to society, may permit these individuals to avoid one of the most devastating experiences of the usual life of the retarded—loneliness (Katz, 1972; Menolascino, 1972). However, marriage must still be viewed as a *possibility* open to the mentally retarded, not a *necessity*. Should marriage be chosen, it must be recognized that support, both financial and emotional, may be necessary from the beginning to maintain the couple's relationship.

Procreation

Considerations regarding the presence of children in the home of retarded parents concern the adequacy of parental care. Like any other behavior, parenting by the retarded ideally requires training, supervision, and environmental and emotional support. To require standards of excellence on the part of those who care for children may be an appropriate endeavor (if standards could ever be equitably evolved), but if these requirements are applied to the retarded parent they should also be applied to the non-retarded parent. Although there is documentation of cases where it has been necessary to remove children from homes where one or both of the parents have been retarded (*e.g.*, Mickelson, 1947; Scally, 1973), this rate should be compared to that of the normal IQ couples of the same socioeconomic class. There may be closer scrutiny applied in a home where it is known that one parent is retarded.

In investigating the percentage of retarded children born to one or two retarded and once-institutionalized parents, it was found that when both parents were retarded, 40% of their children were retarded also. When one parent was retarded, 15% of the children functioned in the mentally retarded range. When neither parent was retarded, the rate was 1% (Reed and Reed, 1965). Therefore, the relative risk of further retardation is much higher among the offspring of retarded parents. In examining the association between IQ and the number of offspring (when childless couples are included in the analysis), it was found that 1) there was no correlation between measured intelligence of the parents and the number of children born, and 2) the retarded had a reproductive rate lower than that of the non-retarded (Reed and Reed, 1965). Although there are exceptions where an individual retarded couple has a large number of children, the average is lower than that for the normal IQ marriage.

The sociosexual model we offer children as they grow up is that of finding a mate, marrying, and having children. Just as we reinforce no alternative models in normal IQ children, we offer no other possibilities to the mentally retarded; yet we are aghast because each young retarded girl, at puberty, wants to have a baby. We do the retarded an injustice by waiting until this desire appears at puberty to remind them of the responsibilities involved in marriage and family. Early sex education may correct part of this deficit. In addition, it might be helpful for the retarded person to be in job training in a nursery, day care center, or kindergarten. This practical training might satisfy the need for children, and might demonstrate that the person is capable of adequately caring for a child.

Sex Education

It is generally accepted that knowledge regarding sexual function enables a person to understand, interpret, and deal with sexual urges more successfully. The mentally retarded, typically, do not possess adequate sexual knowledge (Hall, 1974). In addition, lack of judgment in social situations, characteristic of most of the mentally retarded, makes the deficit even more apparent. Therefore, many feel that sex education is even more important for the person who is mentally handicapped. Parents convey attitudes regarding sexuality in the handling of their child from infancy on, but they may be the most unequipped people emotionally to discuss the topic in a more structured manner. Therefore, if their retarded child is not in a sex education class in school, parents should be encouraged to enroll the child in a class or, if the subject is not being taught in school, to apply pressure to the appropriate authorities so that one will be developed. The program should be a part of the regular school curriculum, taught by the regular classroom teacher every year beginning with entrance into school. It should be repeated each year with increasing complexity, so that by puberty topics such as menstruation, sexual intercourse, venereal disease, and birth control can be understood. Simultaneously with sex education for the retarded, parents should be provided with sex education, along with discussion or therapy groups to handle their emotional reactions to sexual questions proffered by their adolescents. Before the course is begun, teachers will require the same degree of attention to subject matter and attitudes. The initiation of these programs for the mentally retarded has received more discussion and attention than has the evaluation of the methodology used. In order to know the best way to educate the retarded in this area, evaluation must be built into every program.

There is usually little sex education provided to the mentally retarded other than where babies come from and, in the case of females, menstrual hygiene at puberty (Goodman *et al.*, 1971; Hall, 1974). Then, when normal heterosexual attachments occur, parents and teachers somehow are convinced that these persons cannot learn to cope with methods of contraception or decisions about marriage and parenthood. The truth is closer to the statement that the retarded have not been adequately educated in these areas. Only after having so educated them can we possibly say that they cannot understand. Parents must be encouraged to view their retarded child as a sexual being from earliest childhood on, and to view sexuality as a part of the developmental process and not something that can be ignored or eliminated. However, telling the parents that sexuality is a basic right is a gross oversimplification. While it is recognized by many that the mentally retarded have the basic right to sexual expression, and while it is true that sexual expression and marriage enrich the lives of some of the mentally handicapped, it should be pointed out that society does restrict the rights of individuals when those individuals cannot engage in those rights properly. Sexual rights do entail responsibilities. The recognition of these responsibilities is best handled through consistent sex education programs.

GUIDING PRINCIPLES

Some suggestions might be helpful in viewing the sexual behavior of the mentally handicapped.

Professional Contact with the Family of the Retarded

The physician and other professionals in close contact with the retarded and their families should introduce early the topic of sexuality and how it might be expressed by the child, rather than wait for the parent to verbalize fears at the first pubertal sign. Just as sex education cannot be very effective if it is doled out only when questions are asked, physicians cannot wait for questions from parents. The periodical medical checkup should include specific questions directed to the parents about sexual expression, exploration, masturbation and sexual orientation, in addition to an inquiry as to whether the child has asked sexual questions. Any definition of sexuality should include not only activities of an explicit sexual nature but also social derivations of sexuality, such as being attractive to the opposite sex, dressing nicely, wearing appropriate jewelry and makeup, shaving, planning leisure time, and modeling behavior after the prevailing standards. The physician, in so approaching the subject, presents a model that suggests that sexuality for the mentally retarded is normal and part of the developmental process, and at the worst is just one more adjustment problem, as it is for those with normal IQ's.

Normalization

In planning for the mentally retarded, the concept of normalization governs decisions regarding habilitation and education. Normalization means "utilization of means which are as culturally normative as possible (typical or conventional) in order to establish and/or maintain personal behaviors and characteristics which are as culturally normative as possible" (Wolfensberger, 1972). This, in essence, implies the right to live as closely as possible a life typical for the general population. The most obvious implication of this principle relates to decisions about allowing the retarded the enjoyment of sexual expression, including intercourse, marriage, and procreation.

Least Restrictive Alternative

The means employed in the normalization of the retarded should be the least restrictive means available, i.e., why sterilize when a birth control device such as the IUD can be used to control reproduction, or, why not allow marriage, but with contraception, if the couple is incapable of caring for a child? The response of society to sexual expression in the retarded up until several years ago was sexual segregation in institutions or sterilization. Legal statutes prevented marriage in a majority of the states. Now those concerned with the mentally retarded have realized that there is dignity acquired by the retarded in their taking risks in life (Perske, 1972). The United Nations General Assembly and the American Association on Mental Deficiency have drawn up statements delineating what the rights of the retarded should be. Our courts of law have been concerned with litigation pursuing the rights of the retarded. Professionals and parents alike have realized the need to release some power of decision-making to the mentally retarded, while simultaneously realizing, in some cases, the necessity of emotional and financial support.

REFERENCES

Butler, F. 1945. Quarter of a Century Experience in Sterilization of Mental Defectives in California. Am. J. Ment. Defic. 49: 508-513.
Edgerton, R. 1967. *The Cloak of Competence—Stigma in the Lives of the Mentally Retarded.* Berkeley: University of California Press.
Flory, C. 1936. The Physical Growth of Mentally Deficient Boys. Monograph of the Society for Research in Child Development 1 (16).
Fujita, B., Wagner, N., and Pion, R. 1970. Sexuality, Contraception, and the Mentally Retarded. Postgrad. Med. 47: 193-197.
Goodman, L. 1972. The Sexual Rights for the Retarded—A Dilemma for Parents. In *Sexual Rights and Responsibilities of the Mentally Retarded* (M. Bass, ed.). Proceedings of the Conference of the American Association on Mental Deficiency, Region IX, University of Delaware, Newark, Delaware, October 12 to 14.
Goodman, L., Budner, S., and Lesh, B. 1971. The Parent's Role in Sex Education for the Retarded. Ment. Retard. 9(1): 43-46.
Gordon, S. and Green, J. 1972. Sexuality in Courtship, Marriage and Parenthood among the Retarded. Paper presented at the meeting of the American Association on Mental Deficiency, Minneapolis.

Hall, J. 1974. Sexual Behavior. In *Mental Retardation and Developmental Disabilities: An Annual Review*. Vol. 6 (J. Wortis, ed.).

Heber, R. 1970. *Epidemiology of Mental Retardation*. Springfield (Ill.): Charles C. Thomas.

Johnson, A. and Szurek, S. 1952. The Genesis of Antisocial Acting Out in Children and Adults. Psychoanal. Q. 21: 323-343.

Katz, G. (Ed.). 1972. *Sexuality and Subnormality: A Swedish View*. National Society for Mentally Handicapped Children. London.

Kempton, W. 1973. *Guidelines for Planning a Training Course on Human Sexuality and the Retarded*. Planned Parenthood Association of Southeastern Pennsylvania, Philadelphia.

LaVeck, G. and de la Cruz, F. 1973. Contraception for the Mentally Retarded: Current Methods and Future Prospects. In *Human Sexuality and the Mentally Retarded* (F. de la Cruz and G. LaVeck, eds.). New York: Brunner/Mazel.

Mattinson, J. 1973. Marriage and Mental Handicap. In *Human Sexuality and the Mentally Retarded* (F. de la Cruz and G. LaVeck, eds.). New York: Brunner/Mazel.

Menolascino, F. Sexual Problems of the Mentally Retarded. Sexual Behav. 2(11): 39-41, 1972.

Mickelson, P. N. 1947. The Feebleminded Parent: A Study of 90 Family Cases. Am. J. Ment. Defic. 51: 644-653.

Mickelson, P. 1949. Can Mentally Deficient Parents Be Helped to Give Their Children Better Care? Am. J. Ment. Defic. 53: 516-534.

Mosier, H., Grossman, H., and Dingman, H. 1962. Secondary Sex Development in Mentally Deficient Individuals. Child Dev. 33: 273-286.

Perske, R. 1972. The Dignity of Risk and the Mentally Retarded. Ment. Retard. 10(1): 24-27, 1972.

President's Committee on Mental Retardation. The Six-Hour Retarded Child. A report on a Conference on Problems on Education of Children in the Inner City. August 10-12, 1969. Airlie House, Warrenton, Virginia.

Reed, E. and Reed, S. 1965. *Mental Retardation: A Family Study*. Philadelphia: W. B. Saunders.

Scally, B. 1973. Marriage and Mental Handicap: Some Observations in Northern Ireland. In *Human Sexuality and the Mentally Retarded* (F. de la Cruz and G. LaVeck, eds.). New York: Brunner/Mazel.

Tarjan, G. 1971. Sex: A Tri-Polar Conflict in Mental Retardation. Unpublished manuscript.

Wolfensberger, W. 1972. *The Principle of Normalization in Human Services*. National Institute on Mental Retardation, Toronto.

chapter

15

In May 1970 the cover of Time magazine featured Dr. William Masters and Mrs. Virginia Johnson. They had just published their text on treating persons with "sexual dysfunction." These two words, an addition to medical vocabulary, were short-hand for impotency and premature ejaculation in the male, and nonorgasmic or painful intercourse in the female. The book became a best seller.

The treatment technique and results of Masters and Johnson were unparalleled. The treatment program lasted but 2 weeks. The overall success rate averaged about 80%. This success rate, coupled with the estimate that 50% of all married couples experience some form of sexual dysfunction, sparked an unprecedented interest in sexual therapy. One result has been that increasing numbers of patients are seeking help for sexual problems in the context of their general medical care.

The next three chapters present three approaches to the treatment of sexual dysfunction. One is by a male clinician working as a solo therapist who describes his approach to communicating with couples. Another is by a female clinician working solo describing treatment strategies with low income patients, some without partners, and the third is the classic model of the intensive 2-week male-female co-therapist approach as practiced at the Reproductive Biology Research Foundation, founded by William Masters and Virginia Johnson.

Editor

Treating Sexual Dysfunction:
The Solo Male Clinician

CLARK E. VINCENT, Ph.D.

Every physician is a *consultant* in sexual health—whether by choice or default. The physician may ignore the patient's comments and questions in these areas or even explicitly state that he knows nothing about and does not treat sexual problems. However, if he then makes no effort to refer the patient, he is in effect serving as a consultant by having communicated to the patient either that such problems are unimportant or that they have no relation to health.

My intent most certainly is not to add yet another area to the many fields over which physicians are already spread too thin or expected to be all things to all people. But the practice of medicine is consumer-oriented, and patients will continue to perceive their physicians as consultants in times of sexual stress. It is to the physician's advantage, therefore, to perform this role as effectively and expeditiously as possible within the context of his medical-practice model, that is, the procedures, communication techniques, and sequential questions he uses in the practice of medicine.

There are physicians who state, "My patients *never* ask questions about sex." Such a statement could be an indication that the physician's medical specialty is totally unrelated to any illness which might influence or be influenced by sexual behavior and attitudes; but it is questionable that such a specialty exists. More likely, the statement indicates one of two possibilities: 1) that the physician's medical practice is on such a specialized and quantitative basis that he has no contact with patients as individuals, or 2) that the lack of comfort in discussing sexual problems is so apparent that patients "protect" the clinician, and themselves, from embarrassment by not asking questions.

It is not surprising that the physician frequently tries to avoid dealing with problems in the sexual area of patients' lives. Often there has been the warning that the treatment of sexual problems is highly complex and requires special knowledge, skills, and techniques. Therapists and professionals in the field of human sexuality tend to present to audiences of physicians their most complex and involved cases, which require referral and long-term treatment. In what follows, my emphasis is on ways in which the physician can help reasonably healthy couples resolve sexual problems and improve their sexual health.

USE OF THE MEDICAL-PRACTICE MODEL

Office expenses and the number of patients to be seen generally preclude the physician's use of a "50-minute hour." Such time is impractical on a regular basis unless one becomes a full-time specialist counseling in sexual and marital problems. By serving as a consultant in a way that is consistent with the medical practice model, however, one can be helpful to the patient within several 10- to 15-min. periods.

The medical-practice model for obtaining the patient's medical history emphasizes: 1) clear and comfortable communication between the physician and the patient, 2) a logical sequence of questions relevant to the presenting problem, and 3) follow-up questions to clarify the meaning of the patient's answers to earlier questions. For example, if the patient complains of pain with urination, only a novice medical student would write, "complains of pain with urination" in the medical record and ask no further questions. Unfortunately, such comments as "complains of pain with intercourse" are frequently found in medical records, with no evidence that additional questions were asked.

By training and experience, the physician becomes comfortable (and thereby makes the patient feel comfortable) in asking specific questions about whether the pain with urination is greater when the bladder is full or empty and at the beginning or the end of voiding; whether there are differences in the pain at various times of the day; the history and duration of the pain, and so on. The questions are highly specific and relevant to the patient's presenting problem.

In the area of sex, however, the physician departs from his medical-practice model when he asks such vague and general questions as, "How is your sex life?" or, "How is sex?" or perhaps, "How is your love life?" Such questions usually appear to bother the patient, not necessarily because they deal with sex, but because they are so nonspecific as to be unanswerable. The patient would undoubtedly be just as confused and uncomfortable if the physician were to ask, "How is your urinary life?" or "How is your defecation life?"

When a female patient complains of "pain with intercourse," follow-up questions should be as specific and comfortable as those which would be asked about pain with urination:

"Is the pain greater in some coital positions than in others? What exactly does the pain feel like? Does it occur at the moment of insertion? With thrusts? With the absence of foreplay? With the weight of the male? With lack of pleasure?"

Much has been written during the past decade about the inability of physicians to discuss sex with their patients. But there are many physicians who have a high degree of comfort and skill in consulting with patients. Some obstetricians, in particular, have developed the art of using an ongoing consultant dialogue that continues from one 10-min. office visit to the next during pregnancy and the postpartum period, and for routine gynecological checkups. Over a period of years, many hours of dialogue can be carried on in 10-min. sessions.

Future developments will undoubtedly make the taking of a complete sexual history a more efficient and economical process than at present. For now, it seems to me that the physician is wise to follow basic medical procedures of asking specific questions that are logically related to the patient's presenting complaint or comment.

"MY HUSBAND DOESN'T SATISFY ME"

Some of the foregoing points can be illustrated with a composite case history which reflects one current presenting complaint of female patients: "My husband doesn't satisfy me sexually." But first, a relevant digression.

Reasons for the Increasing Frequency of This Complaint

Twenty years ago, the couples who came to me for marriage counseling included a sizeable number of husbands complaining of sexually unresponsive wives. Within the past several years this pattern has been reversed; now, I see more wives lamenting about husbands who do not satisfy them sexually. Some of these wives have been married 2 months; others, 20 years. For the latter group, the publicity given the results of the Masters and Johnson research has made it more acceptable and respectable for females to seek the sexual pleasure that they may have been denied in prior marital years.

One reason for the failure of some women over 35 years of age to experience sexual pleasure with their husbands relates to a general difference between males and females in their physiological conditioning with regard to orgasm—a difference that may be less applicable to those under 30. The male often starts self-stimulation very early; he is goal-oriented, and his purpose is to achieve orgasm. A female may begin at 10 or 11 to hold a boy's hand and may get her first kiss soon thereafter. During several years of dating in high school and college, she is increasingly stimulated sexually and often reaches the "plateau stage." But traditional societal *mores* have warned that this is as far as a "nice" girl should go. By the time of marriage, she may have had 5 or 10 years of training to get excited to a point and then say, "That's far enough."

Experiencing an orgasm is something like learning a new word: both involve a synaptic connection—an impulse passing or "jumping" from one neuron to another. By the time you've heard the word 12 times, you have a nice groove between the two neurons. The male comes to marriage with a beautiful groove for his orgasmic synapse; in many cases the female has no such groove—and to make such a connection more difficult, she has built in a physiological dam. Most males can reach orgasm quickly. All too frequently it was a case of "Wham, bam, thank you ma'am." The bride was lucky if she reached the plateau stage. This may be why Mark Twain purportedly observed that Niagara Falls was the *second* greatest disappointment to honeymooners.

A Composite Case

The following is a composite case to illustrate ways in which the physician can obtain from and share with the patient relevant sex information. Assume that a female patient married 15 years has indicated directly or indirectly that sexual relations with her husband are not entirely satisfactory.

Doctor: "Would you like to talk about it?"
Patient: "Yes, but I don't know if anything can be done."

Doctor: "Do you enjoy sexual intercourse?"
Patient: "No, not really."
Doctor: "Have you ever enjoyed it or felt any sexual pleasure?"
Patient: "A little maybe when we were first married."
Doctor: "Have you ever experienced an orgasm, a sexual climax?
Patient: "I think maybe; I don't know."
Doctor: "Have you and your husband discussed this?"
Patient: "Yes, *ad nauseam*! He thinks somehow I'm just not normal or something. And I guess I wonder too."

Ideally, at this point the physician would make an appointment to see this patient and her husband together—a procedure followed by an increasing number of physicians who set aside one half-day each week for 30-min. appointments with couples. Often such a joint interview will eliminate the necessity for several future visits by the wife alone. A number of physicians, in the case of a husband who is reluctant to come in, make use of a brief telephone conversation.

Doctor: "I've just seen your wife in regard to her fatigue problem (headaches, colitis, ulcer, etc.) and she mentioned that there has been a rather long-standing problem of very little pleasure and enthusiasm for sex on her part. I think this is something which can be changed, but I need your help and cooperation, since you know her best and are acquainted with the problem. I would like for you to come with her for the next appointment."

Husband: 1. "O.K. I'll be there. Thank you for calling."

Or

2. Well, I don't know what I can do. We've talked it to death and I'm pretty well resigned; but if you think it will help, I'll come."

Or

3. "Let me check my schedule first. I think I'm tied up that day. I'll call you back."

Or

4. "No. I see no point in my coming. I've said and done all I can on this subject. If you can change her, that's great. She only gets mad when I talk about it."

In response number 3, the husband may feel that he is caught off guard and wants time to think it over and perhaps check first with his wife to "find out what she said about him." If his return call is still evasive, the doctor may then simply assume and explicitly emphasize the husband's concern for his wife and his consequent willingness to help, whether it be with a broken leg, a bleeding ulcer, or lack of sexual satisfaction—all of which involve the husband in the treatment process.

In response number 4, the doctor can 1) use the foregoing approach of assuming the husband's basic concern and love for his wife, 2) assume that the husband will not want the doctor to perceive him as callously having no love or concern for his wife, or 3) authoritatively communicate to the husband that without the husband's help treatment will take longer and cost more.

The couple have now come in for their first joint session.

Doctor (to the wife): "You indicated last week that you were not sure whether you had ever experienced a sexual orgasm, or climax. Tell me if you have ever felt somewhat like this." (At this point he inhales six or eight times, each time faster, and then completely relaxes and lets his arms and head sag.)

Wife: "Well, sort of; I have felt the first part."

Doctor: "Explain, please."

(The wife may then inhale rapidly several times and then "tense up" rather than relax; she may even hold her breath. If the doctor is watching the husband's face, he may see the husband's dawning and partial awareness of what it has been like for his wife for 15 years to become sexually excited and be left on the plateau stage. He may also begin to understand why his wife appears to be so irritable the day after any coital activity.)

Doctor: "Let's approach the problem first on a physiological basis." (He then explains a synapse in relation to learning a new word, learning golf, or having an orgasm.) "You also indicated last week that you thought you had some sexual pleasure when you were first married, but now you have little interest in it. I think it is very normal for you to feel no interest in sex at the present time. In fact, it would be quite understandable, given your circumstances, if you even hated sex now."

Husband: "She does! Sometimes she even hates me for it."

Wife: "Not really. I mean I don't hate you; but sex—well, yes, I guess I do."

Doctor: "I think your feelings are entirely normal. Let me explain why,
by analogy. During your first months of marriage—maybe even
for the first year or so—coitus was exciting because you (the
wife) felt just like you did when you were courting and you
reached the plateau stage of excitement.

(Here the doctor may draw an oversimplified diagram to illustrate her plateau and the block created by her physiological
conditioning, taking care to point out that the diagram is only
one of several possible response cycles for the female.)

"After awhile, however, you became aware of somehow being
left in mid-air—excited but frustrated and without completion—
possibly left at either point *A* or point *B* (in Figure 1). If you
will accept the analogy, your experience has been to be teased
with a succulent beefsteak, which was taken away just as you
started to partake of it. Time and time again, you were excited,
then frustrated; excited, frustrated; excited, frustrated. Gradually you learned that the only way to keep from getting frustrated
was not to be excited. Finally sexual intercourse became quite
distasteful to you. Why? Because you not only failed to get the
steak; you had to be present and watch your husband enjoy his
steak (orgasm), while you had none. No wonder you hated sex
after a while! Put yourself through the same kind of conditioning with steak (see it, anticipate eating it, then have it taken
away from you to be eaten and savored by the very person who

Figure 1. Stages of sexual response cycle and potential blocks.

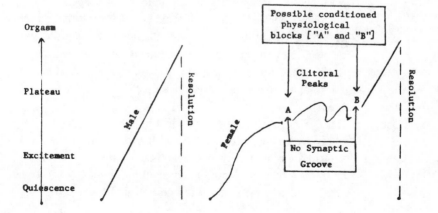

seemed responsible for depriving you of it) and I think you would have little interest in steak, or would actually hate it.

"If what I have described fits your experience, you can see why I think your present lack of enthusiasm for sex, or even dislike of it, is a very normal feeling for you. I think you (speaking to the husband) can also see from the analogy why you are probably quite accurate in feeling that at times she hates you because of sex. Neither of you should blame the other for the tragic fact that each of you has been denied a degree and quality of reciprocal sexual pleasure that was rightfully yours these past 15 years. Instead, blame the myth that human sexuality is not a proper educational subject—the myth that sex is so simple as to be learned naturally."

Wife: "No wonder my mother was so negative on sex. I wonder if she went through her whole life without ever having any real pleasure out of it."

Doctor: "Now, let's focus on the task of how the two of you can help you (the wife) to experience an orgasm. First, you (the husband) will have to guard against being defensive when your wife tells you what feels good and what doesn't. This defensiveness is not peculiar to you; you share it with most men of your generation.

"Why is it so difficult for a wife to tell her husband what gives her sexual satisfaction? If your wife asks you to scratch her back and you comply, she doesn't hesitate to give you instructions: not so hard; now over to the left, under the shoulder blade; slow down. . .easier; over to the center. . .*there*. She can give you six or eight sets of instructions and it doesn't bother you. Why? Because no one ever told you that expertise in backscratching has anything to do with masculinity. Therefore, your male ego isn't threatened, and she can give as many instructions as she wants. But can she give you six or eight different instructions on how to give her sexual pleasure?"

Wife: "I couldn't give him two."

Doctor: "This is largely because males in our society learn at a very young age to equate *masculinity* with *knowing all about sex*. In elementary school, you can hear two or three boys talking: Jimmy is a sissy; he doesn't know anything about *it* (sex). To be a real boy, to be masculine is to know all about sex.

"This indoctrination puts the adult American male in a box and keeps him from learning about female sexuality. To learn something about a subject, you have to admit you don't already know everything there is to know; but for the male to admit there's something about sex he doesn't know is for him to question his own masculinity.

"Remember that your wife is the only one who can tell you what feels good to her. When you feel you are becoming defensive, try telling yourself that she is only suggesting how you can scratch her back."

Wife: "He's really good at that."

Husband: "Yes, because I know you'll scratch mine."

Doctor: "Let's consider more specifically what you feel or experience when your husband caresses the clitoral area."

Wife: "Mainly, it's very irritating."

Husband: "She doesn't like it very long."

Doctor (to the husband): "Imagine your wife taking about one-half square inch area at the head of your penis and rubbing her finger or hand across that one small spot as rapidly as possible." Frequently the husband will wince or even pull back his pelvis at the thought; but it helps him understand why it is irritating to his wife when he locates and focuses almost exclusively on a very small area of the clitoral hood. "The whole general area of the clitoris is laced with sensitive nerve endings, and this is why you need to be guided by what she suggests, even down to the pace and direction of your caressing." This explanation is another example of specificity of counseling, in contrast to general advice such as, "Caress the clitoris."

"Also (to the husband) we need to be specific about how much time is spent in caressing the clitoris. The irritation resulting from concentrating on too small an area probably means you have not caressed the clitoral area more than 5 to 10 min. and that she is 'trying too hard' to respond before it becomes irritating."

Wife: "Yes, that fits; but what else can you do? I know he is getting excited and that very little is happening to me, so why not have him come in and get it over with?"

Doctor: "That makes sense, given your experiences up to now. But we are trying to change a physiological response to which you have

conditioned yourself for nearly 20 years—getting up to the
plateau and then stopping at point *A* (in Figure 1). Specifically,
it means sessions of 20 to 30 min. of caressing with fingers, lips,
tongue, in a way that is not irritating—*and* savoring the caressing
rather than trying to produce an orgasm. By analogy, the meals,
plays, or walks you enjoy the most are those you savor in process, not those you desire only to complete."

Some wives who indicate that they have never gone beyond the conditioned physiological *A* (in Figure 1) may be helped by the following explanation:

Doctor (to the wife): "Since you have not yet experienced an orgasm, it is
possible that sometimes you are very close to a climax but then
suddenly become tense because of fear that you will urinate if
you let yourself go. The sensation produced by sexual excitement can be quite similar to the rather exquisite pain which can
accompany a very full bladder. Thus, the brain may be trans-
lating an unfamiliar message (approaching climax) to a familiar
message (very full bladder)."

I cannot defend the neurological accuracy of this simplistic explanation,
but many couples to whom I have offered it have subsequently reported that
it helped the wife to ignore the fear of urinating and to continue through to
orgasm. In a few cases, the wife has reported, "I did dribble a few drops the
first time, but I wasn't too embarrassed and it's never happened again."

In other cases, further information given to the husband may be what is
needed. Sometimes the husband who is trying to help his wife enjoy a more
complete sexual response is concentrating so hard on the techniques of
satisfying her, or on delaying his own orgasm, that he inadvertently or purposely dampens his own ardor and passion; and in such cases the wife may
find it difficult to respond fully unless she feels that her husband is as fully
aroused as she. Not knowing what she might say or do in the moment of
orgasm, she may want him to be as "gone" or "lost" as she—not a spectator
observing her from the sidelines. Women reflect this feeling sometimes in such
comments as, "Don't ask, just take me!" or "Don't diddle or tinker with me,
just let me feel your uncontrollable desire for me!"

HELPING COUPLES TO CHANGE SEXUAL ATTITUDES
AND PRACTICES

At first the couple may feel that dwelling on the specifics and techniques of lovemaking makes it seem contrived, mechanistic, and awkward. *It is.* The first time a beginning golfer tries to keep his elbow straight when he hits the ball, it feels awkward and mechanistic too; that's part of the learning process—but he gets through that phase. Couples who assume that their lovemaking must always be impulsive, spontaneous, and romantic have forgotten that "artful" dancing, piano-playing, or golfing can come only after considerable practice and many "mechanical movements" in the early stages of learning.

The Need for Patience

Every physician needs a supply of examples and analogies that will help him illustrate specifics rather than quote generalities when counseling patients. The following analogy is one which can be helpful for the spouse who is impatient with the married partner's slowness in changing a given attitude concerning sexual behavior.

Doctor: "If you are attending an international meeting of 100 people in some European country and want to find out which of the 100 were the 10 attending from the United States, request the maitre d' to serve pie for dessert. When the pie is served with what we regard as the "back side" Δ toward the diners, the 10 people from the United States most likely will turn the piece of pie around ∇ to begin eating from the pointed end of the wedge."

Wife: "What's the point?"

Doctor: "Within the next 24 hr (as well as any time either of you feels impatient with the other's reluctance or slowness to change an attitude in the sexual area), try eating a piece of pie by starting from what we regard as the back side. I think you may experience some such feeling as 'It doesn't taste as good,' 'It doesn't feel right,' or 'It isn't natural.'

"If you do experience any of these feelings (even while telling yourself, 'It isn't evil; it's all right to eat it this way'), you will better appreciate the strength of 'culture' — the accustomed ways of eating, behaving, or thinking. And if it takes you a little time and repeated attempts before you feel comfortable with such a relatively simple change as eating a piece of pie from a different angle, you will have more patience with the time required for you or your spouse to feel comfortable in making changes in the emotionally loaded area of sexual behavior."

Upside-Down Thinking

The compartmentalized, and even upside-down, nature of our thinking about sex is frequently reflected when the couple wants to talk or ask about caressing the genitals with the mouth or tongue. The wife may state that she enjoys her husband's oral caressing of the clitoral area, but that her enjoyment is marred by feelings that it is "dirty" or "unnatural." It is, of course, quite unsanitary — primarily because of the high bacterial count in the *mouth.* With normal hygienic practices, the genitals can be the cleanest parts of the body. It is the mouth which is unsanitary; yet couples rarely think of osculation, or oral kissing, as unclean. Nor does the female think it unclean for a male to kiss her hand, which has handled money that has gone through the hands of a few hundred other people with various germs.

The notion that oral-genital contact is "unnatural" also reflects a lack of logic. In the areas of food, wine, and the arts, for example, we compliment people who enjoy a wide range by calling them gourmets or connoisseurs. The greater a person's capacity to enjoy variety in color, in food, in music, and in the decorative arts, the more we admire that person for having developed and utilized all of his or her God-given senses. In the sexual area, however, we turn this concept upside down—regarding as "unnatural," or even "perverted," sexual practices designed to appeal to *all* the senses and to afford pleasure by a variety of means.

"CLITORAL PEAKS" AND FEMALE ORGASMS

That the sexual response cycle varies considerably among women has long been noted, more recently by Masters and Johnson who also have described variations for the same woman at different times. In Figure 1, I differentiated between 1) "clitoral peaks," followed by slight resolution to the plateau stage, and 2) an orgasm which exceeds the clitoral peaks in "height" or intensity, followed by a major resolution phase similar to that of the male. I base this pattern on the following composite of experiences reported by wives and confirmed by their husbands: 1) "I can experience several peaks with clitoral stimulation, but only one big one which usually, but not always, comes with insertion." 2) "After one or more peaks with clitoral caressing, my (vaginal) opening is so tight (small) that he has to enter carefully; but after a big (full, complete) one, my opening is so big he feels lost inside if he hasn't already come." 3) "After one peak I may want more peaks or want him inside for the big one; but after the big one, even if I haven't had any peaks, I'm through, relaxed, and just want to rest or go to sleep." 4) "The good feeling from the peaks is fairly local. I know where it is coming from, and I can have several of these in succession. But the big one involves me all over, from stem to stern, and I have no inclination to repeat it till I've rested for a while."

Since the publication of some of the findings of Masters and Johnson in popular magazines, an increasing number of couples are discussing the meaning of 1) "multiple orgasms," and 2) the wife's awareness of a difference, in kind or degree, between her response to clitoral stimulation and her response to insertion. In some of these discussions the wife may add that the number of her clitoral peaks can easily exceed her husband's number of orgasms, but that she does not desire to exceed his frequency with what she may refer to as her "full," "complete," or "insertion" orgasms.

Few of these couples have read the two books authored by Masters and Johnson, and sometimes their questions and discussions reflect some of the incomplete if not distorted ideas conveyed in magazine articles. The questions and observations of some women about their own sexual responses are in the context of the very old debate concerning the "clitoral" *vs* the "vaginal" orgasm—a debate sparked by Freud's view that the vaginal orgasm was a more "mature" sexual response.

It is not my intent to rekindle this debate. It is my intent: 1) to report a female sexual response pattern which some couples have experienced and can describe in detail; 2) to accept their experience and descriptions as *real* for them; and 3) to note the implications for the physician working with a couple who, in reference to the diagram shown in Figure 1, experience a block at point B: although clitoral stimulation by self or partner enables the wife to experience one or more clitoral peaks, she still feels unsatisfied and never (or rarely) experiences any response to insertion. Thus, the physician's early question to the wife as to whether she has ever experienced sexual orgasm may, in some cases, need to be followed by more specific questioning as to whether the wife's answer refers only to clitoral peaks resulting from caressing of the clitoral area, or whether it includes an orgasmic response with insertion.

COITAL FREQUENCY AND THE
PROBLEM OF STATISTICAL NORMALCY

Other factors are involved in the foregoing composite illustrative case, but *all* of these factors are rarely involved in any one case. The physician who heeds the medical-practice model is well aware that "sex problems" like "respiratory problems" can have many symptoms and causes. Medical training and medical-practice experience also warns of the danger of being bound by statistical definitions of normalcy when treating the individual patient. The normal body temperature of 98.6°F. is a statistical average that certainly does not fit everyone, and rarely fits the same individual throughout a 24-hr. period. Similarly, the "normal frequency" of two or three coital unions per week is a statistical average produced by couples who, at one extreme, find satisfaction in having coitus three times a day, and by other couples who find satisfaction in a frequency of once or twice a month. The "problem" of coital frequency, in which one spouse blames the other for "abnormally" frequent or infrequent desire for sex relations, may be created when the accusing spouse accepts as "normal" a statistical average which fits few individual couples and rarely fits any one couple over a 3-month period.

The ludicrousness, as well as the danger, of enslavement to "the average" is readily apparent from the following story, borrowed from the statisticians. The physician may find that this story, or a similar one, provides perspective for couples who are too much influenced by "the average" when rearing children, assessing their coital frequency, or counting their orgasms.

Two statisticians in the Allies' front-line trench during World War I observed a German soldier rushing toward them with rifle cocked and bayonet fixed. When the first statistician fired his bullet went to the right. The second statistician fired and his bullet went to the left of the onrushing German. The two statisticians dropped their rifles at this point and embraced each other happily—because"on the average" they had him.

chapter

16

Treating Sexual Dysfunction:
The Solo Female Physician

DIANE S. FORDNEY SETTLAGE, M.D., M.S.

There is nothing unusual about solo treatment of marital relationships or an individual's problems which include sexual dysfunctions. Both psychotherapy and marriage counseling programs, usually supervised by one therapist, include sexual function. However, they generally have not included specific treatment plans for sexual dysfunction. Approaching sexual dysfunction as a primary problem, rather than as one secondary to other relationship or individual difficulties, is a recent development.

The team therapy approach utilizing a male and female therapist working with a male and female sexual unit (couple) is currently the ideal and most advocated method for treating sexual dysfunctions. The advantages of team treatment are primarily those of modeling by the therapy unit for the dysfunctional unit, same sex identification and opposite sex reaction for each member of the treated unit, and the synergistic advantage of two experienced counselors. The disadvantages of team therapy can be both arrangement and treatment related. One must remember that modeling and identification transference can be negative. If the therapy team contains one weak and one strong member, they may work well together, but for the patient identifying with the weak therapist and from the non-egalitarian model presented to the unit, problems may be intensified. If stylistic, social, interactional, or emotional differences exist between the team treatment members, these too may be transmitted to patients as a negative model. Certainly formation of teams requires considerable self-with-other learning, training, and objective evalua-

213

tion of the team's effectiveness. Counselors and physicians are trained for autonomy and rarely relate intimately as professional peers. Thus, we are faced with difficulty in establishing a complementary, effective, egalitarian team.

Considerations of practicality are real. Finding female cotherapists is a serious problem. Women physicians are rare, regardless of interest. Male physician therapists then look to women with nursing, psychology, sociology, or other educational backgrounds to serve as cotherapists. Again, physician contact with these groups is not fostered by the medical community and, when it exists (as with nurses), is rarely on a peer level. Although these problems of identification, availability, peer-relatedness, informational and attitudinal differences, and individual personality can be overcome, they pose formidable obstacles.

Additionally, the demand for sexual counseling far outweighs the supply of competent therapists. Restricting sexual therapy to team treatment thus reduces by half the available services of professionals. Whether this is justified in terms of higher success or reduced numbers of visits per unit is not known. For the physician who is unable or unwilling to do full-time sexual counseling but can work at least 8 hours per week in the area, the problems of scheduling with a cotherapist can be monumental. The alternatives are then single therapist treatment or no treatment. Medical and other professional services remain grossly inadequate for all levels of society in utilization of dual-sex team therapy for patients with sexual dysfunction. Utilization of dual sex therapy teams for individuals, groups of same-sexed individuals, or groups of mixed-sex individuals is largely unevaluated but these situations might be equally or more suitable for the solo therapist.

Within the medical profession, women are fairly well represented in the field of psychiatry and many have dealt extensively with sexuality. However, within psychiatry, sexual problems have been treated largely by analytical and insight-psychodynamic techniques which exert their effects secondarily, if at all, on sexual dysfunction. For other medical specialists, educational programs, counseling skills and training settings have been virtually nonexistent.

Women are becoming physicians at a higher rate than ever before, with a four-fold increase in the last 5 years. To reach proportions equivalent to the female population will require a 10-fold increase and is within the realm of probability; thus, the need for consideration of their role in sexual counseling. This chapter is primarily for their hopefully burgeoning numbers.

Do solo female sex therapists face problems that solo male sex therapists do not? The basic assumption would seem to be that they do. "Men and women do not relate well to women as authorities." "Men relate to women as potential lovers (conquests); women to women as potential rivals." "Men and women are not receptive to intimate discussions of sex with women therapists because of social sex-role stereotyping." Certainly these typical comments may be overriding considerations for some patients, but they also exist in reverse for male therapists. Such considerations probably do exist to some degree in all patients but are easily surmountable and may even be catalytic to the progress of the sexual unit or individual. The major difficulty with such assumptions is their effect on the potential therapist herself because of her social sex role conditioning. An apt analogy would be genital examination of opposite-sexed patients early in medical training. Male students examining women are concerned about sexual anxiety (their own), and being identifiable as crass beginners. Yet they do not express concern about the appropriateness of themselves as males examining women. Female students are often primarily concerned about the appropriateness to the patient (and themselves) of women examining men. They are much less concerned about their own sexual arousal or beginner's status. Physicians become accustomed to having access to other peoples' bodies, performing surgery, and dealing capably with desperate disease—all of which engage powerful socialization taboos. The interested female physician can similarly become capable and comfortable in sex therapy.

I do sex therapy alone with individual women and groups of women who either have no current sexual partner or whose partner has chosen not to participate. Such situations are not rare, nor are they unique to female therapists. Obviously treatment must accommodate itself to the absent partner but is often successful in terms of the patient's goals. When the partner becomes available, he or she is introduced to conjoint techniques if necessary. I also do couple therapy alone and with cotherapists in a training setting. Because I am a female gynecologist most patients referred are "female-problem-identified." However, the occurrence of male partner dysfunctions is high and therapeutic approaches must include their management.

PATIENT REACTIONS TO A SOLO FEMALE THERAPIST

Women have responded immediately with strong positive identification in initial (individual) interviews simply because I am a woman. This is a significant advantage which should not be understated. However, it must be modified in dealing with a couple to avoid male isolation. Attempts of patients to develop female-female comraderie must be discouraged and immediately opened to the male partner. The dialogue and flow of affect is appropriately between the couple via the therapist.

If men evidence discomfort in the initial (individual) interview, the possibility of inhibition produced by dealing with a female therapist should be supportively confronted at that time so that it can be evaluated and granted permissibility. The remainder of that interview usually progresses well. An opposite reaction, occurring in conjoint sessions, may be a positive affect which excludes the female partner. This too must be confronted by including the woman and directing the positivity to her. Usually, such a male reaction occurs when he feels threatened by or hostile to his partner. The therapist must always remain secondary to the unit cohesiveness. Direction and reinforcement of positive feeling, intermediary control and restatement of negative feeling, and introduction of new ideas, form the basis of the therapist's role in couple management. Your ease in discussing sexual detail comfortably, and sensitivity to the feelings of each partner can then provide a model for the couple that is topic and person related, rather than male or female related.

MANAGEMENT OF SEXUAL DYSFUNCTION

Treatment of sexual dysfunction, as discussed here, is related specifically to sexual symptoms and encompasses techniques from several disciplines. Informational, attitudinal, and physical education of patients is a major part of the process. Development of communication skills for sexual disinhibition is another. Physical and emotional conditioning exercises in self-assertiveness, sensory awareness, receptivity, and transmittability of sexual feeling are combined with the protective transference of responsibility from patients to therapist. Psychodynamics can be identified by the physician, and insight often occurs, but the emphasis is on the current behavior and feelings. Therapeutic results are grouped in terms of both the alleviation or elimination of the symptom, and improvement in acceptance of self and partner.

Sexual dysfunction treatment is not primarily psychotherapy or marriage counseling. It deals with those factors that currently affect sexual satisfaction. It is possible to resolve sexual dysfunction and have the marital relationship either improve or terminate. It is also possible to accomplish only the identification of serious relationship problems from which the sexual relationship will not recover until the total relationship does. The therapist must here decide if she wishes to become a marital counselor or to refer that unit and resume sexual therapy at a later time. It is extremely uncommon to see no relational problem in patients with dysfunction. Assessment of these problems is mandatory to determine if sexual counseling would be of benefit. Where discord is not bitter, or alienation of the couple is not pronounced, sexual therapy often provides the communication tools to reduce marital problems. Occasionally, psychopathology can be identified in one or both partners which requires psychotherapeutic intervention. In this case, the rapport you have established may be instrumental in utilization of a referral.

What is the management plan for treatment of sexual dysfunction? There are specific physical techniques applicable to the nature of the complaint which have been well stated elsewhere. For the county hospital clinic population with which I work, it is rarely if ever possible to begin therapy at that point. Lower educational level, adherence to the double standard in sex roles, accepted male-female inequality in the relationship, absence of prior exposure to counseling, and severe financial limitations require modification of techniques. For the female in the unit this means training in self-assertion and self-pleasure. For the male, it means learning to share involvement and responsibility with his partner. For both it often begins in solitary activity which is verbally communicated, and nonthreatening physical contact.

The first interview consists of three parts in couple treatment—a joint interview, and a separate interview with each partner. Often the order is female, joint, male interview; or female, male, joint interview. Obviously the concern in beginning with an individual interview is that the partner feels he is already excluded. In my practice, however, usually the woman has identified herself alone as having a problem, or her partner has told her she does; and she is not at all convinced there is help for her. She is reluctant to involve him until she has been told she is a suitable candidate for treatment, and the therapist confirms the importance of their mutual involvement. She then has the therapist's support to say "Since we are both unhappy, we need to work together" or "It is necessary for you to help me, will you?" Let me stress how difficult this can be for some patients, and that insistence on a joint initial interview may result in repeated appointment failures. If her partner refuses, she is a candidate for individual treatment both in terms of identifying her relationship needs and in terms of working on sexual and communication skills.

When the male partner agrees, there is a positive effect relating to the expression of commitment, willingness to share, and relief of isolation. This is intensified in the initial joint interview where both people speak together of the problem as they see it, and the attendant feelings they can express. I do not obtain a complete history at that time. Rather, the couple is given a detailed history form which they fill out separately at home. It obtains consistent information, allows the patient ample time for reply, saves physician time and can be referred to as necessary throughout treatment.

The purpose of the individual interviews is to gain access to feelings the patients are reluctant to express in front of their partner or behavior they have not confided. Privacy is respected but strong encouragement to relate or modify current behavior is mandatory. Premarital coitus unknown to the partner may or may not be relevant to treatment. However, extra-relationship coitus which is almost always suspected by the partner, and not honestly confronted by the couple early in the treatment period, is invariably associated with treatment failure. Sham orgasm in the dysfunctional woman must be first eliminated and then confronted before therapy can succeed. Lack of love for or relative indifference to a partner is also a prognostic sign of failure, unless dealt with and modified. Usually the therapist can facilitate the sharing of such information by the third or fourth conjoint session. If not shared, mutual sexual relearning and communication cease in the next few sessions. Other relational problems are often obvious by then to the unit and the sexual therapist must decide whether to continue as marriage counselor or to refer. That decision is made in light of the clinician's background skills, interest and time. Often the suggestion of referral, followed by another appointment, will result in overcoming the impasse, or patient agreement that referral is appropriate.

After the three-part initial interview, complete physical examinations are scheduled for both partners. Who does the exams is not critical, provided the physician is informed of the history and knows how to do a sexual problem-oriented examination. Organic causes of dysfunction are relatively rare but may more frequently be contributing factors. There is a positive effect in therapy if the treating clinician performs the examinations. However, if the problem is identified as primarily female, and the male partner has evidenced reluctance to participate or anxiety about a female therapist, I will ask if he prefers a male physician for the examination.

The second joint session focuses in more detail on sexual techniques, experience, and feelings (sensory and emotional) during sexual encounters. Patients are instructed to refrain from coitus, and their concerns about this discussed. They are given educational material about sexual response and behavior to read together, and instructed to spend 15 min. each day lying nude, holding and talking to each other. Verbal expression of how this feels while it is occurring is stressed—both positive and negative. Nonsexual physical demonstration of affection at other times is encouraged—touching, smiling, stroking, hugging, and kissing. Both partners are instructed to initiate. Physical sexual arousal stimulation is forbidden. If either partner interprets physical contact as sexual, he or she is to state that verbally to the partner. Couples who have reacted positively to this with comfort and pleasure during a week's trial may be appropriate for the sensate focus exercises which are described below. Units which avoided or reacted negatively are not. Concerns about each other's reactions must be explored and understanding established. The therapist must attend to expressions of fatigue, lack of privacy, too much to do, and resentment. All are ways of avoiding intimate contact which is nonsexual in nature. It is often necessary to plan time and place with the couple so it is established daily. The feelings, anxieties, and reactions to each exercise or assignment often form the nucleus of discussion in the next therapy session.

In the third session instructions are given for self-body examination (nude in front of a mirror) and detailed self-genital examination (using a mirror and comparative picture). The latter includes the introduction of fingers into the vagina and attempts by women to palpate their cervix. The focus is on learning, comfort with all of their body, and recognition of anxiety. During the same period the couple together learn body massage for relaxation and take turns in its administration to each other. Again the emphasis is on giving and receiving physical pleasure that is totally nonsexual and is relaxational rather than anxiety producing.

Massage is then followed by holding. Discussion of body image (self and partner) and physical attitudes or habits which each find attractive or repellant for themselves and their partners occurs in the next session. Patients then explore each other's bodies with verbalization of reactions and playful, fun elements all emphasized. This follows reciprocal massage. Separately they explore modalities of tactile stimulation, all nongenital, with emphasis on sensory appreciation and anxiety recognition. Patients are also instructed in breathing and muscular techniques to apply when anxiety occurs. This includes deep breathing and attention to the relaxation of the muscle groups. Genital self-stimulation techniques including use of mechanical appliances for production and recognition of sexual responses and arousal patterns are next taught. Women learn Kegel's (1952) exercises, repetitive contraction and relaxation of the pubococcygeus muscle, to increase cognitive awareness of perineal and pelvic activity. Mutual nongenital stimulation for pleasure is initiated with the passive partner (recipient) first instructing, then receiving pleasure, and anxiety is communicated as directly as possible. The mutual program, even though only one partner may be "dysfunctional," makes both participate equally. From this point, the principles described in the book of Masters and Johnson, *Human Sexual Inadequacy* (1970), are followed in general principle.

Throughout, attitudinal and educational discussion is continued, with graduated use of explicitly sexual diagrams, photographs, and films for their educative, communication enhancing, inhibition lessening, and sexually arousing properties. Romantic and erotic fantasy is encouraged and shared. Fantasy can be useful in both anxiety reduction and arousal enhancement. Destructive relationship actions and reactions are identified and modification instituted. Goals are always pleasure, comfort, and mutuality with coital expectation and coital outcome de-emphasized.

The general outline given above is followed for most patients. However, the emphasis and specifics of treatment are highly individualized to each couple or patient. Some require more time in self-acceptance and allied anxiety reduction techniques. Others require more effort and time in the elimination of destructive interactions and the development of those which are enhancing. Disparities between the members of a couple may be great, as with a man who has great difficulty in assuming the passive role while his partner has become fully assertive. For some, certain techniques must be eliminated or greatly modified to avoid the creation of value or personality conflict. An example of this would be the devout Roman Catholic and techniques of masturbation. Patients always provide the framework within which the therapist must work. The goal of sex therapy is that which patients determine. The clinician's role is to assist in utilizing all and only those tools which suit that goal.

REFERENCES

Beck, A. T. 1970. Role of Fantasies in Psychotherapy and Psychopathology. J. Nerv. Ment. Dis. 150: 3-17.

Cooper, A. J. 1969. Some Personality Factors in Frigidity. J. Psychosom. Res. 13: 149-155.

Ellis, A. 1960, *The Art and Science of Love*. New York: Lyle Stuart.

Hastings, D. W. 1963. *Impotence and Frigidity*. Boston: Little, Brown and Co.

Holroyd, J. 1970. Treatment of a Married Virgin by Behavioral Therapy. Obstet. Gynecol. 36: 469-472.

Jones, W. J. and Park, P. M. 1972. Treatment of Single Partner Sexual Dysfunction by Systematic Desensitization. Obstet. Gynecol. 39: 411-417.

Kegel, A. J. 1952. Sexual Functions of the Pubococcygeus Muscle. West J. Obstet. Gynecol. 60: 521.

Lazarus, A. A. 1963. The Treatment of Chronic Frigidity by Systematic Desensitization. J. Nerv. Ment. Dis. 136: 272-278.

Lazarus, A. A. 1971. *Behavior Therapy and Beyond*. New York: McGraw-Hill.

LoPiccolo, J. and Lobitz, W. C. 1972. The Role of Masturbation in Treatment of Orgasmic Dysfunction. Arch. Sex. Behav. 2: 163-171.

Madsen, C. H. and Ullmann, L. P. 1967. Innovations in Treatment of Frigidity. Behav. Res. Ther. 5: 67-68.

Masters, W. and Johnson, V. 1970. *Human Sexual Inadequacy.* Boston: Little, Brown and Co.

Ullmann, L. P. 1965. *Case Studies in Behavior Modification.* pp. 243-245. New York: Holt.

Weitzman, B. 1967. Behavior Therapy and Psychotherapy. Psychol. Rev. 74: 300-317.

Wolpe, J. 1958. *Psychotherapy by Reciprocal Inhibition.* Stanford: Stanford University Press.

chapter
17

Treating Sexual Dysfunction:
The Dual-Sex Therapy Team

MAE BIGGS, M.S.
RICHARD SPITZ, M.D.

Possibly, as many as 40% of sexual dysfunctions in marital interaction could be prevented, or be treated successfully, by physicians in practice, were they thoroughly informed about sexual psycho-physiology. However, the physician who is informed relative to human sexual response, and who could, or would take the time to treat sexual dysfunction, must recognize limitations of expertise, particularly in interpreting and representing the opposite sex in this most vulnerable mode of communication in interhuman interaction, sex.

This chapter describes the potential of the dual-sex therapeutic approach. In any sexual dysfunction, there is no uninvolved partner. No male distress lacks female contribution; the converse also pertains. Furthermore, since no male can ever fully comprehend femaleness (nor the converse), we endorse therapy for sexual inadequacy by both a female and a male serving as cotherapists.

Therapy of inadequate pair-unit (couple) interaction at the Reproductive Biology Research Foundation is directed to development of a functional interaction between two people, each an individual to be supported in the given relationship. This implies a healthful total interactive communication pattern within the relationship, with focus on the vital component of any such intimate couple interaction: sexual functioning. For purpose of definition, "sexuality" encompasses the totality of communication modes by which gender identity is expressed. Humans express and communicate "sexuality" in various ways including dress, physical characteristics, and timbre of voice. They also do so in sexual function. "Sex," a natural psychophysiological function, is just one way in which sexuality is communicated. Sex is the most intimate and vulnerable form of interhuman communication, both psychological and physiological. To treat a pair-unit relationship for the sexual component alone would be overemphasis on but one factor of the way in which sexuality is communicated. In order, then, to therapize effectively, attention must be paid to all the ways in which the pair-unit interacts, including the sexual. This therapy is best interpreted when the female therapist supports and represents the female, and a male therapist interprets the male.

The concept of therapy at the Reproductive Biology Research Foundation embodies several fundamental features. The therapists must direct attention to principles of interpersonal communication of sexuality in pair relationships. These principles imply that each person in the relationship has an obligation to represent self and to do so by taking the risk to make his own needs known first. The same principles of communication apply in sexual function.

Despite folklore and tradition to the contrary, the double standard (in which the female is, supposedly, intuitive in social communication, and the male, supposedly, intuitive in sexual function) falls short of reality. In a functional pair-unit relationship, each member must be vulnerable to desires, wants, needs and requirements, at any time, in any place, under any circumstance of partner interest, whether in communication of sexuality, or sex, to the partner. *Effective* sexual activity involves two individuals, operating on an equalitarian basis in the relationship—enjoying self "with" the partner, rather than doing something "to" or "for" the partner.

Were therapists to define and direct patients on the bias of their own personal credos or by any other imposition of the therapists' personal guidelines, it would constitute disservice to the unit in therapy. If the therapists feel they cannot treat the situation within the core-value systems that the patients present, they are well advised to acknowledge the fact and to refer to another authority.

The Foundation therapists see a spectrum of pair-unit distresses which range from those in which sexual communication is not too impaired, but social communication (shared feelings) is ineffective. Also seen are couples whose social communication remains intact despite almost complete breakdown of sexual interaction. Most couples present to the Foundation because of specific sexual distress. Inevitably, however, this or these dysfunction(s) spread to the inclusion of social communication breakdown. This phenomenon can be expected because the most vulnerable form of interhuman communication, sex, has failed. Therefore, in most instances of therapy, the spotlight focuses on the sexual functioning of the pair interaction. The relevancy of this form of communication then extends to total communication.

In this societo-cultural scene, it is usually more difficult for the male to express his fears, needs, and wants in the social component of the relationship. Males are socialized to be problem solvers in everyday life. Therefore, for many males, sexual functioning is the outlet for a release of either the day's frustrations, or celebration of the work-a-day triumphs. For the female, the converse pertains. In this societo-cultural schema, the female places higher priority on the total security of the relationship. For her, sexual function implies a total socially communicative atmosphere, involving her own private or public aspirations, the home, the family's hierarchies, and the children. Physiologically, she is the more versatile of the two sexes in sexual capability. Socially, culture has imposed suppression of her sexual expression. Conversely, males have been imprinted with the social picture: "tough, dispassionate, un-feeling."

MALE DYSFUNCTIONS

I. Premature Ejaculation The male ejaculates so rapidly after vaginal penetration that the female has little or no (50% probability) opportunity to achieve orgasmic return, assuming orgasmic facility.

In premature ejaculation, a technique for gradual abatement (3 to 6 months) of ejaculatory urgency has been documented as effective. This technique requires the cooperation of the female partner. While premature ejaculation is a male dysfunction, it eventually gives rise to the female's distress. Therefore, prolongation of ejaculatory control is to the female partner's advantage.

To enhance ejaculatory control, the female will incorporate the squeeze technique on the penis during sexual activity, and *not* just prior to ejaculation. The female partner uses the pad of her thumb on the anterior surface of the erect penis and the index and middle fingers contraposed to the thumb— the index finger just above and the middle finger just below the coronal ridge of the penis. She squeezes firmly for 3 to 4 sec. and, after quick release, explores other parts of his body before returning to specific penile stimulation. This technique needs to be incorporated three to five times prior to vaginal intromission throughout each opportunity of penile play for about 3 months, at 50% of opportunities for at least another 3 months, and then, whenever lack of opportunity exceeds 3 to 5 days, depending on age.

The neurophysiological mechanism of male onset of ejaculation is unknown (as also is true of onset of labor or female orgasmic response). However, it *is* known that the squeeze technique prolongs ejaculatory control if, and when, it becomes a natural and easy part of sexual play, rather than a clinical exercise.

Commonly the male who has a long history of premature ejaculation is accompanied by a female who is unable to experience orgasm ("situational nonorgasmic return") with intercourse. Although she may be orgasmic by other modes, layers of resentment accumulate because of her interpretation of being "used" by the male, or a "second best" way to "get the job done."

Therapy for such couples must include much unlearning. Both partners are unknowledgable about the physiological nature of premature ejaculation and cannot fully comprehend how sex can be so bad when all other communication is so good. Therapy for such dysfunction directs attention to the detail of effective pair-relationship communication.

II. Secondary Impotence. The male has been successful in achieving and maintaining an erection adequate for either heterosexual or homosexual penetration in the first, or the first 1,000 plus opportunities, but fails to do so currently in at least 25% of opportunities.

Secondary impotence is the next most commonly reported male sexual distress. It is also almost surely avoidable when males and females understand the realities of sex as a mutually interactive male/female phenomenon. Undoubtedly in our day, the most prominent cause of secondary impotence is aging. Yet, at onset, such distress is noth a dysfunction but a natural part of the aging process.

Unfortunately, all too few people, including physicians or other authorities consulted, are aware of the natural history of sexuality in the aging despite the fact that information on this subject has been available since 1964. As a physiological phenomenon of male aging, frequency of need to ejaculate, rapidity and tonicity of penile erection, volume of ejaculate, and force of expulsion all gradually decrease.

Certain characteristics are common to both males and females with aging. Again, because culture has dictated that sexual function implies penis in vagina, far too many males, unable to rise to the occasion at a given opportunity, are programmed to feel (and the female partner and medical authority agree) that they are over the hill and that a rocking chair is the most sensuous pleasure to be expected. As a consequence, sex is out of context. The failure to achieve and maintain an erection at any and every opportunity means failure as a male, even to the female. For too many current sexagenerians, and older, this concept has eventuated in avoidance of sexual function for 20 years or more. All this is based on misconcept and misinformation.

The second most common cause of secondary impotence is a long history of premature ejaculation. Like the aging male of this day, the premature ejaculator, misinformed to believe that the male must provide adequate duration of vaginal containment to accomodate the reputedly slower female responsiveness, is given to know, by the female partner, that he is not "getting the job done." He begins to try too hard. Not uncommonly the distress is not made a matter of contention until the female realizes that the youngest child is becoming self-sufficient and soon there will be just the two — man and woman. Then she wants the sexual fulfillment that her assigned responsibility for family rearing previously denied her. He is repetitively struggling to maintain interest and praying for long enough erective and ejaculatory prolongation to fulfill his woman. By reason of "working at it" erections adequate for sustained mounting become fewer and farther between.

The third leg in the causative triad of secondary impotence is alcohol or other anesthetic drugs, usually beginning in middle age. While a dram of alcohol may relax sexual inhibition for either male or female and serve to enhance sensuous awareness, its use to enhance sexual "staying power" all too frequently bombs out...figuratively and literally.

For the male, fear of his not being able to "get the job done" is of paramount importance in secondary impotence. It is difficult for the female partner or cotherapist to fully appreciate the intensity or depth of the impotent male's erective insecurity.

The female plays her role in the evolution of male impotence because she commonly assumes there is something wrong with *her* if the male is no longer at the ready for needs. She still believes (and male "authority" is inclined to reinforce the concept) that now that children are reared, he should begin to take care of her as first priority, whether or not prior casting has placed her in the role of mother, cook, or a mere sexual recipient, and him in the role of "giver of security."

Therapy of secondary impotence requires much unlearning and reorienting for both male and female partners. Beyond the time required to dispel misinformation, misconcept, myth and taboo, effective reconstitution requires spelling out the psychophysiological factors of total communication which are applicable to the specific breakdowns of the pair in therapy.

III. Primary Impotence. The male has never achieved or maintained an erection adequate for either heterosexual or homosexual penetration in his lifetime.

This male dysfunction is quite another matter. Whereas secondary dysfunction arises from the ashes of misinformation and the recriminations of both sexual partners, primary male impotence usually arises out of self-fear, usually not sexual-partner imposed or enhanced. There is an exception to this which will be discussed subsequently in the consideration of vaginismus in the female.

Therapy in such circumstances requires infinite patience on the part of the female partner and the therapists. Obviously, this distressed male would not apply for therapy had he no interest in trying to establish his own sexual capability, both for self and partner. Each element of his and his partner's sexual reserve, the physical and laboratory examinations and the interactive patterns, socially and sexually, of both will dictate the therapists' therapeutic approach.

IV. Ejaculatory Incompetence. The male sexual dysfunction of ejaculatory incompetence may be a "never happened," or may have occurred at least as a one time phenomenon of intravaginal or intra-anal ejaculation. This distress may be either primary or secondary. In the male who has never ejaculated intravaginally, there is commonly a history of strict religious orthodoxy, much concern that sexual functioning is dirty or sinful, and that seminal fluid and the vaginal environment are contaminated.

The female partner may be quite pleased with the long-maintained erection without ejaculation but the unit may come because ejaculatory incompetence constitutes a problem, if conception is desired.

The secondarily ejaculatory incompetent male may present a history of some event in which he either perceives the female partner's vagina as "contaminated" by another male partner, or has intense fear of pregnancy and has used withdrawal as means of birth control. Another precursor is prolonged use of ejaculation control as a means of "punishment" of the female partner for real or imagined offenses. Beyond these, anesthetizing levels of alcohol or drugs, including amphetamines, may so desensitize sexual excitation that sensuous feelings necessary for ejaculation are not achieved.

Parenthetically, like premature ejaculators, the ejaculatory incompetent male also may become secondarily impotent for the same reasons, namely, he is not completing the standardized requirements of "appropriate" sexual function and becomes a fearful spectator.

Therapy of ejaculatory incompetence, which is a relatively rare complaint in Foundation experience, consists primarily of pointing out the origins of the distress to both partners. Beyond this, self or partner manipulation just to the point of ejaculatory inevitability, prior to inserting the penis, is advised. Getting the first intravaginal ejaculation is not uncommonly a long process. Beyond the first, however, progress is rapid.

FEMALE DYSFUNCTIONS

Orgasmic return is a natural psychophysiological component of female sexuality. Culturally, however, the female has been imprinted to think socially first and, only at a later age than males, sexually.

The female is taught at an early age to repress her sexuality. Many are socialized to believe that the genital area is associated with uncleanliness since the vagina is located between the urinary orifice and the anus. For example, it is common for the male to be praised by mother and father alike when he learns to hold the penis and urinates standing up, for being "such a big boy." The female is generally instructed that she, upon urinating, must wipe her genitals with tissue, must not let her hands touch the area in the process, and immediately following such action, must wash her hands. Great stress is placed to keep the genitals clean, untouched by human hands, and "guarded." In essence, the female is taught not only not to touch or permit herself to be touched in this area except for "clinical duties," but also not to acknowledge feelings in the genital area as pleasurable. Societo-cultural imprinting imposes that "decent, respectable females" do not honor their sexual feelings. Denial of self as a sexual being is infused within the value system of many females.

Another variant of the socialization process with regard to maleness and femaleness is that surrounding pubescence. Nocturnal emissions in the male signify that masculinity has been attained. The male can now *possibly* impregnate the female. For the female, first menstrual flow also signifies that she can *possibly* become impregnated. However, these body fluids, granted the difference in both quality and quantity of function, take on societo-cultural evaluative aspects with reference to sex. The ejaculate becomes a symbol of masculine prowess; the menstrual flow is unfortunately, frequently labeled as the "curse" or the "sickness."

Small wonder that the natural physiological response in the female is *culturally* repressed. But physiological research shows that the female is potentially more versatile sexually.

I. Primary Nonorgasmic Return. The female has never perceptively achieved (or identified as such) sexual tension release (orgasm) by any means, whether via self-manipulation, partner-manipulation, or intercourse.

The primary nonorgasmic female has been permeated with "shall nots," either overtly or covertly. Emphasis is placed on "not to touch," "not to enjoy being sexual," "sex is the male's prerogative," "she should serve and please." These "shall nots" internalized from family, peer group, or religious orientation, with the consistent stress to the female of negatives associated with the broad spectrum of sexual communication, inhibit or distort development of an effective sex-value system.

II. Situational Nonorgasmic Return. The female has been able to identify sexual release by one, or several varieties of stimulation techniques such as masturbation, partner manipulation, mouth-genital stimulation, or, less frequently, intercourse, but not by all modes.

Random Non-orgasmic Return. The female has been orgasmic possibly by both manipulative or coital stimulation, but, *rarely*, during the sexual opportunities of the specific couple.

The situational or random nonorgasmic female has been orgasmic at least part of the time. She may have been orgasmic, situationally, in intercourse, by masturbation, by partner manipulation, or by any combination. It could be so historically infrequent to be categorized as "random." The historical development may contain elements similar to that of the primary nonorgasmic female. Particularly, she may incorporate the idea that sex is the male's prerogative and it is what he will *do to* or *for* her that will make "something" happen, such as orgasm.

The therapy process for the nonorgasmic female, whether primary, situational, or random, will vary from individual to individual and from couple to couple. Common to all distresses, however, is a history of removal of sex from its natural context with consequent fears of failure to perform adequately. Orgasm as a natural psychophysiological phenomenon is emphasized in the therapy process. No attempt is made to teach the female how to be orgasmic in therapy. There is no specific formula applicable to all women for attaining orgasm. The female is permitted the opportunity, often for the first time, to explore and experiment with varieties of sensuous feelings, sensations, and stimuli with her partner. Emphasis is placed on the nonproductivity of the "observer's role." She is advised to avoid any attempt to make sexual feelings, lubrication, or orgasm happen and to take the necessary risks to experiment and explore feeling levels on a moment-to-moment basis.

Concomitant with the sharing of physiological information of sexual responsivity with the nonorgasmic female and her partner, integration of this knowledge with their independent sex value systems is suggested; myths and misconcepts are dispelled and each partner is encouraged to assume responsibility for personal sexual responsiveness. This approaches a philosophy of sex as a natural psychophysiological process. Therapy provides each partner the opportunity to innovate, creatively, alternate means and varieties of stimuli which will accumulate sexual feelings necessary for orgasmic release.

III. Vaginismus. The female has involuntary contractions of the ordinarily expansive pelvic-supporting muscles in the outer one-third of the vagina to the extent that penile penetration becomes extraordinarily uncomfortable for the female, or frequently, impossible, for the male.

The female and, consequently, the male partner thus affected, frequently come to therapy because the marriage is not consummated. Often the male has been in psychotherapy for years because he is "primarily impotent." Usually the female has been of the belief that sex is a 'no-no' unless in marriage. Usually she has visited at least one professional authority who failed to recognize the involuntary spasm of the vaginal entry. Hence it is assumed that nonconsummation is the male's problem. The fear is established.

Therapy is uniformly effective if "vaginismus" is purely a female distress. Dilation of the vaginal opening with use of graduated dilators, and steroid replacement as indicated, is a simple process. However, because the male usually is "afraid of hurting her," therapy directs attention to the interactive phenomena while the couple uses the vaginal dilators in privacy.

DISTRESSES OF EITHER MALE OR FEMALE

I. Sexual Aversion. This phenomenon of disinterest in sexual functioning occurs in both females and males. The diagnosis implies fundamental facts. Aversion may be directed to the marital partner only and/or to any specific type of sexual activity. Sex, uniquely, of all natural physiological processes, can be voluntarily set aside for a lifetime if celibacy is a choice. Natural phenomena during dream states, *e.g.,* nocturnal emissions in the male, or orgasm in the female, may intercede. But with aversion, negative psychophysiological factors in the couple's interaction may dictate that sex becomes importanly unimportant, and leads to absolute avoidance. Thus, all feelings, including sexual, are voluntarily or involuntarily suppressed, negated or denied. Once again, it is imperative that appropriate questions are asked of patients during the initial interview sessions, in order to determine those factors which contribute to the aversion.

Surprisingly, aversive response to sexual function is a relatively simple therapeutic entity. Many adversive sexual couples have had sexual function so much out of natural context that therapy evolves as though each partner were waiting for the therapists to offer them permission to be sexual.

There may have been such dysfunction as dyspareunia, vaginismus, non-orgasmic return, premature ejaculation or male impotency which, either in present or past pair-unit interactions gave rise to sexual avoidance. But, most frequently, they need little more than the intensive concern of cotherapists who give each the encouragement and "permission" to represent self, both socially and sexually.

II. Dyspareunia. THis condition is painful intercourse (which can occur in both males and females). This rare cause of disharmony is of such multifaceted origin that it cannot be clearly spelled out in this brief chapter.

In the female, the more common physical factors include a retroverted uterus, the breakdown of the broad ligaments supporting the uterus ("universal joint syndrome"), vaginitis, or inadequate steroid replacement therapy, during or after menopause.

In the male, prostatitis due to chronic congestion as an end result of "withdrawal" for birth control, or any other "need" to halt ejaculation, may give rise to a heavy prostatic sensation, aching of the testes, or a sharp discomfort at the distal end of the penis.

It cannot be stressed too strongly that the therapy of any couple's dysfunction or discord must be tailor-made for that particular relationship. Once having ascertained how each of the individuals has developed his/her value, or nonvalue, of self, and the significant features of the evolution of their system of sex values, therapy simply and nonjudgmentally mirrors back to each individual, and to the relationship, those components of interaction. Then, by means of sharing candid, accurate information relative to the individuality of sexuality and pair-unit sexual functioning, and stressing the need for individual self-representation in the relationship, therapy directs attention to alleviation of these discordancies which have frustrated effective sexual interaction.

REFERENCES

Masters, W. H. and Johnson, V. E. 1966. *Human Sexual Response.* Boston: Little, Brown and Co.
------, *Human Sexual Inadequacy.* 1970. Boston: Little, Brown and Co.

chapter

18

Pornography in the classroom? During the past few years human sexuality courses have increasingly utilized explicitly sexual films. Why? Is this for purely sensational reasons, or are there educational benefits which follow?

To remain unaffected by these visual materials is difficult. Their impact is alleged to catalyze dialogue on patterns of sexual behavior. And, when they display sexual conduct previously not experienced or witnessed, it is asserted that they provide new information. The educator's hope is that the physician's own sexual growth will, in turn, permit more comfortable and effective patient counseling.

Strategies for integrating the range of available erotic films into programs of instruction in human sexuality are varied. They constitute a cutting edge in contemporary health science teaching. This final chapter describes these materials, some methods for incorporating them into medical curricula, and provides support for their educational value.

Editor

Sexually Explicit Media in Medical School Curricula

HERBERT E. VANDERVOORT, M.D.
REVEREND TED McILVENNA, M. Div.

We live in a media-oriented society in the midst of an information and communications "explosion." With the increasing public acceptance of explicit sexual content in legitimate art forms and media of all kinds, it is not surprising that the use of graphic materials has gradually become an accepted and valuable element of education in human sexuality.

RATIONALE

The two most important reasons for using graphic materials in courses in human sexuality are to communicate information and to assist the student in developing a useful and accepting attitude concerning his or her own sexuality and the sexuality of others.

The use of graphic media as a means of communicating information is relatively easy and less valuable than the use of such materials to assist in developing an effective clinical attitude and personal frame of reference. Our experience has shown that the major impediment practitioners suffer in doing sex counseling is not primarily due to a lack of information (although many are not accurately informed). Rather, it is a result of guilt and self-recrimination over their own sexual fantasies and experiences and anxiety about the sexuality of others. This results in their attempting to compensate for these conflicts by the misuse of professional authority to impose self-comforting myths on patients. Many practitioners "deal" with sexual problems by simply denying that they exist.

An example of how explicit graphic media can be most useful is the area of homosexuality. Here social condemnation and the practitioner's own conflicts or fears conspire to render the clinician less effective in helping that 10% of the population which is homosexual. Explicit films showing the sexual patterns of homosexual couples who love each other have proven invaluable in increasing the awareness and acceptance of the students viewing them. While the films do eliminate some of the mysteries concerning the mechanics of *how* homosexuals relate physically, (facts), they are much more important in terms of the "meta message." The meta message to the student is: "See, you can look at this. What homosexuals do is not much different than what heterosexuals do. Homosexuals care for each other just like others and you do not have to be afraid of them."

Students generally report a lessening of anxiety about homosexuality following viewing homosexual content films and develop a freer attitude about learning more about homosexuality. Admittedly, the same effect could be achieved by an inspirational lecturer or a well done legitimate play or movie. However, the graphic film which is produced specifically for educational purposes has the advantage of being brief, inexpensively duplicated, and easily included with other similar materials to form part of a course. Here we have used the "topic area" of homosexuality to illustrate the rationale for the use of graphic media. Next, consider the rationale for use of media in a more general way.

Graphic media can be used to create a variety of educational experiences in which the effect of the whole is greater than the sum of the parts. By utilizing existing graphic, explicit media in relatively large numbers and in a planned sequence, it is possible to prepare the student to be more receptive to serious consideration of emotion-laden areas to be presented later. First, materials of a neutral sort are presented, followed by materials designed to "desensitize" and relieve anxiety. Through a process such as this, *early* in the course, graphic materials are of value in helping the student to become more receptive to later potentially emotion-laden topics of greater importance. A number of medical schools and other educational institutions are presently using graphic sex educational materials in this way. In various combinations, "neutral" materials are shown first to put human sexuality in an historical context and to show that human sexuality has been a concern of creative artists throughout history. Then, materials are introduced to "desensitize" the students, either by presenting an overload of visual sexual materials, or by presenting emotion-laden materials followed by small group discussions. Still later, materials can be used for instruction in specific content areas.

MATERIALS AVAILABLE

The types of media available vary from conventional instructional materials on how to obtain a sex history through sexually explicit films illustrating sexual behavior of a wide variety. Similarly, the methods of use vary from the occasional use of one or more films, to illustrate a specific topic or stimulate discussion, to the use of many and multiple media in a programmed process. This will be described later.

Because new materials are constantly being produced by many educational centers, we will not attempt to list them all here. However, the major resource centers most likely to be informed concerning materials available are the following: The National Sex Forum in San Francisco which pioneered in the production of explicit films and media for sex education for professionals; the Sex Information and Education Council of the United States (SIECUS) in New York which has pioneered in developing, cataloging, and annotating sex education materials for wide use; The Center for the Study of Sex Education in Medicine in Philadelphia which has pioneered in the development and cataloging of curricula and materials used in medical schools; and the Institute for Sex Research in Bloomington, Indiana (Kinsey Institute) which has extensive references and material covering the entire field of human sexuality. The largest distributor of graphic sex education materials is Multi Media Resource Center in San Francisco. MMRC is the distributor of National Sex Forum produced material and also distributes films produced by independent film makers.

Films available consist of art films, a collection of commercially produced sex action films, and documentary films produced specifically for educational purposes. The art films vary from a prize-winning "erotic" film depicting a close-up of an orange being peeled in such a way that an erotic effect is produced, to films of montages of nude individuals to films of female genitals. The collection of commercially produced sex action films consists of materials dating from the mid-1920's. These depict most forms of sexual behavior which has been filmed for the commercial market and are used generally for their historic value and in a desensitization process.

Most of the documentary films distributed by Multi Media were produced by the National Sex Forum, specifically for educational purposes. In all the National Sex Forum films the "actors" are volunteers who agreed to be filmed as their personal contribution to the fund of knowledge about human sexuality and sexual behavior patterns. Films commonly used include several illustrating masturbation and masturbation fantasies, methods of sensual massage, patterns of shared sexual experience—both homosexual and hetero-sexual—a film on the squeeze technique for the treatment of premature ejacu-lation, on the sexual patterns of the physically handicapped, the sexual patterns of a woman in late pregnancy, and several rap sessions including discussions on women's sexuality.

METHODS OF USE

While any of these materials can be used alone and have educational value, we have found the use of several films, particularly in a planned sequence, to be more valuable. We have also found that the use of two or three films, side-by-side, simultaneously, has distinct advantages. First, more material and images can be presented in less time. Second, a greater variety of behavioral patterns can be presented in less time. Third, a greater variety of behavior can be simultaneously compared. For example, if three documentary films on masturbation are viewed simultaneously the viewer is impressed with the in-dividuality of the behavioral pattern.

A specific value of using films side-by-side is illustrated by the case of the film of the rap session where individuals with spinal cord injuries are dis-cussing how difficult it was for them to convince themselves and the medical profession that they were capable of sexual activity. When this film is pre-sented side-by-side with an explicit documentary of a couple where the male partner is a partial quadriplegic, the combination of the two films is a more impressive experience.

The most refined and comprehensive use of graphic media of all kinds which has been developed is the method called Sexual Attitude Restructuring (SAR). This was developed and evaluated over a period of 8 years by the National Sex Forum in consultation with experts in educational theory and particularly programmed learning methods. The process has been used ex-tensively in the Program in Human Sexuality at the University of Minnesota and by the Human Sexuality Program at the University of California, San Francisco.

SAR is designed to give the audience a basic background in human sex-uality and to assist persons taking the course to become more aware of their own sexual feelings and attitudes, and to be more accepting of the sexuality of others. This, in an intense brief period of time. The course lasts from 12 to 16 hr. and is given on consecutive days.

Elements of the SAR process are as follows:

1). *Endorsement.* a) Giving permission to look at, experiment with, study and learn about sexuality and particularly one's own sexuality; b) presenting sex as a natural and positive part of life in the broadest sense.

2). *Information.* What people actually do sexually, how they feel about it, how their bodies respond, how sexual expressions vary, what happens at different age levels, and how people deal with family planning.

3). *Masturbation.* How people get in touch with their own sexual responses and fantasies, myths surrounding masturbation, therapeutic uses of masturbation, and varieties of masturbatory experience.

4). *Homosexual Experience.* A form of shared sexual expression; misconceptions, historical perspectives, current attitudes, behavior, and variations.

5). *Desensitization–Resensitization–Exploration of Myths.* Helping people to recognize and accept their own fantasies and the fantasies of others by graphically presenting a broad range of explicit erotic material; sensitizing people to their own sexual preferences and aversions; disconfirming myths and distorted conceptions by presenting authentic behaviors and encouraging people to respond to them.

6). *Comparison of Male and Female Expression.* Implications of the differences in socialization, physiological and behavioral comparisons, responsibility for one's own response.

7). *Sexual Enrichment.* Broadening one's range of fantasies, emotional responses, and behavior.

8). *Cultural expression of sexuality.* How sexuality permeates our culture and is presented symbolically and directly in the arts, music, and media.

9). *Therapy.* Specific methods which can be used to overcome sexual dysfunction and to anticipate and prevent future dysfunction.

10). *Specific Problems.* How the physically or mentally disabled and other minorities are sexually disadvantaged for social and cultural reasons and ways in which these problems can be alleviated.

Although the SAR process may be used in a wide variety of ways and over varying periods of time, a typical course follows:

The audience assembles at six in the evening, and while the group is convening, slides of erotic art are being shown, two at a time, at 8- to 10-sec. intervals. A sound tape is running simultaneously in which the speaker is discussing some of the contradictions and problems faced by our society in sexual matters. An amusing set of slides depicting the biblical prohibition against using sexuality is then presented and the course introduced. A series of art films and fantasy films is shown to put the audience at ease and to lead the audience gradually toward the presentation of more explicit sexuality.

Films illustrating masturbatory patterns are then shown on multiple projections up to three at a time. This is followed by a presentation called "Fuckarama" which is intended to desensitize the audience to a wide variety of sexual materials. Here there are multiple projections of commercially produced sex action films, of four to eight at a time, for an hour. These films depict almost all forms of sexual behavior which have been recorded on commercial film and in approximately the proportion in which this behavior occurs in contemporary society. This experience is intended purposely to overload the senses and exhaust the audience's fears of viewing explicit materials. Then the audience is resensitized with documentary films depicting loving, tender sexual communication, and one or two light-hearted art films which conclude the evening.

During the next day, in various sequences, content areas are presented with films that are appropriate to the area, generally two at a time, with a minimum of lecturing and, depending on the audience and intent of the course, varying amounts of small group discussions. Content areas include shared sexual experience including homosexual, heterosexual, and bisexual patterns, the human sexual response cycle, some aspects of male and female sexuality, sexual enrichment, sex counseling, cultural aspects of human sexuality, and special sexual problems of the physically handicapped.

Ideally, since the SAR course is an art form as well as an educational process, the elements should be given in contiguity. However, the course and the media are adjustable to a variety of curricula requirements. For example, at the University of California, San Francisco, students taking a required course, "Human Sexuality in Medical Practice," go through the evening process as described, followed by 3-hr. lecture and seminar meetings weekly for an academic quarter, during which the rest of the content and materials are presented, and small group discussions held. The important educational principle here is that the evening session, including the sensitization, is preparatory for the presentation of more clearly content-oriented material.

Because individuals who take the course often undergo personal reassessment of their own sexuality and sexual attitudes, we prefer that students attend accompanied by their "significant other." In fact, we believe that in any educational experience where explicit graphic sexual material will be used it is important to have a mixed-sex audience, if at all possible. While the course can be done in an auditorium or classroom setting, because the audience is required to experience the process as well as to learn, we have found that a comfortable setting which avoids the classroom or academic mood is valuable.

Results of the Use of Graphic Media in Sex Education

In evaluating the effectiveness of the use of sexually explicit media we have relied on two sources:

1. Data gathered from persons who have been exposed to graphic media in courses given by the National Sex Forum.
   Over a period of 7 years approximately 30,000 persons have been through these courses.
2. Information supplied by the Multi Media Resource Center, which distributes the materials developed by the National Sex Forum, as to how many institutions are using graphic sexual materials and for what purposes.

The National Sex Forum chose eight categories to evaluate. As shown in Table 1, these were: 1) books of photographs and drawings, 2) tapes, 3) slides of erotic art objects, 4) historic and current sex action films, 5) fantasy films, 6) multi-media approach, 7) setting of the room, 8) talking about sex.

Seven hundred and thirty-nine women and 1,126 men were asked to respond to each of the categories on the basis of whether it had helped them understand their sexuality and the sexuality of others. We asked the participants whether or not they agreed with the three basic assumptions of the National Sex Forum (Table 2). We asked the individuals what their personal reactions were to watching the specific types of sexual activity (Table 3).

Follow-up assessments were also conducted. A majority of medical students reported, 1 year after the course, that they had been helped in talking about sex with their patients and also with discussing *general* medical areas. As for physicians and counselors who took the course, over three-fourths reported they were helped in discussing sex with their patients as well as topic areas not directly related to sexuality. No participants reported detrimental effects.

Another method of evaluation of explicit sexual media has been to document the number of educators presently finding graphic materials helpful and further the number purchasing material for use in the education process.

Multi Media Resource Center provided this information. MMRC's records show that more than 1,300 institutions in the United States are using graphic sex material in their education programs. Their records also show that over 5,000 individual practitioners, counselors, and educators have purchased or

TABLE 1

	Greatly Helped %	Helped %	Neutral %	Detracted %	Greatly Detracted %	Don't Know %	No Answer %
Books of photographs and drawings-Females (N=739)	11	39.1	37	4.3		4.3	4.3
Males (N=1,126)	18	55	19	3		2	3
Tapes (N=739)	35.7	41	14.3	3.6	1.8		3.6
Males (N=1,126)	30.6	48.7	17.4	2.5			0.8
Slides of erotic art objects-Females (N=739)	12.5	53.6	25	3.6		5.3	5.3
Males (N=1,126)	14	58.7	19.8	5	0.8		1.7
Historic and current sex action films-Females (N=739)	47.3	38.4	5.9	2.5		2.6	3.3
Males (N=1,126)	58.3	36.3	3.8	0.8			1.8
Fantasy films-Females (N=739)	46.4	32.2	8.9		1.8		10.7
Males (N=1,126)	55.3	35.5	4.2	0.8			4.2
Multi media approach-Females (N=739)	52.7	36.8					10.5
Males (N=1,126)	62.2	32.4					5.4
Setting of the room-Females (N=739)	56.5	37	8	3		2.2	4.3
Males (N=1,126)	48	40					1
Talking about sex-Females (N=739)	64.8	24.4	8.1	2.7			4.3
Males (N=1,126)	42.9	52.4	3.6	1.1			1

TABLE 3
Reactions

	Aroused	Disgusted	Interested	Shocked	Curious	Disinterested	Informed	Happy	Uncomfortable
MOVIES OF: *Heterosexual Intercourse*									
Male (Rank ordering):	1	7	2	8.5	3	8.5	4	5	6
Female (Rank ordering):	2	9	1	7	3	8	4	5	6
Oral-Genital Sexuality									
Male (Rank ordering):	1	6.5	2	8.5	3	8.5	4	5	6.5
Female (Rank ordering):	2	7	1	9	3	8	4	6	5
Female-Female Sexuality									
Male (Rank ordering):	4	7	1.5	9	1.5	8	3	5	6
Female (Rank ordering):	5	7.75	2	7.75	1	7.75	3	6	4
Male-Male Sexuality									
Male (Rank ordering):	5	7.5	2	9	1	7.5	3	6	4
Female (Rank ordering):	5	8	1.5	7	1.5	6	3	9	4
Group Sexuality									
Male (Rank ordering):	2.5	7	1	9	2.5	8	4	5	6
Female (Rank ordering):	3.5	7	1	8	2	9	3.5	6	5
Sexuality Being Forced on Another Person									
Male (Rank ordering):	7	3	2	6	5	7	8	9	1
Female (Rank ordering):	5.5	2	3.5	7	3.5	8	5.5	9	1

TABLE 2
National sex forum basic assumptions

	Agree		Disagree		Don't Know	
	N	%	N	%	N	%
1. The most significant factor in sex education is that sex can be talked about casually and nonjudgmentally.						
Asked of 1,865 males/females:	1,841	95.8	8	1.4	16	2.8
2. Individuals should be allowed meaningful exposure to a realistic objectification of the range of behavior into which their own experiences and those of other humans fall.						
Asked of 1,865 males/females:	1,846	97	9	1.6	10	1.8
3. The person who teaches, counsels, or gives advice (regardless of professional qualifications) should have a low burden of sexual guilt feelings so as to be of service to others rather than serving his own needs.						
Asked of 1,865 males/females:	1,857	98.6	4	0.7	4	0.7

rented graphic material during the past 3 years. Of additional interest is the observation that of those who ordered material, over three-fourths ordered more.

FUTURE DIRECTIONS

The use of graphic media in the education of medical students and other professionals should increase and become more sophisticated in the future. Media will be produced illustrating a much wider variety of patterns of sexual behavior, and increasingly for specific purposes such as the films already available on the spinal cord injured.

Another trend will be graphic materials produced for self-help and patient educational purposes. These will include video cassettes which a physician can give to his patients either for use in the office or to take home. Similar educational media and materials will be produced as closed loop movie films and sound-sync slide projector systems. We expect that these materials will not only increase the effectiveness of the professional but will also decrease the amount of counseling time required and so cut the cost of health care delivery.

Epilogue

These divers chapters have not covered new areas of human sexuality. The topics have affected the lives of every patient (and our own). Regrettably, they have been largely ignored within the traditional teaching and practice of medicine.

Who among us, as clinician or patient, can remain untouched by considerations of pregnancy control or termination, intercourse during pregnancy, the mentally retarded child, the adolescent with different sexual ethics than his or her parents, the post-heart attack male with anxieties over reinstituting sexuality, the woman reluctant to undergo a pelvic exam, the accident victim with spinal cord injury worried that sexuality is no longer possible, the homosexual patient or colleague, and the couple whose sexual relationship is not all they had hoped for?

Human sexuality is a medical specialty in the sense of other areas of health care. Like other specialties, it cuts across biological support systems and receives significant input from emotional support systems. Like other specialties, there is a factual underpinning rooted in basic science, paced by empirical clinical knowledge, and tempered by individual human considerations.

Medical science will continue to change with the relentless evolution of technological hardware and biochemical surprise. Basic human sexual functioning may be essentially unalterable, but modifications will continue in practices, attitudes, and problems.

Human sexuality is uniquely convoluted. It is the life force necessary for continuation of the species; its excesses can also endanger the species. It is the focal point of concern by both the secular and the religious, each exerting forces of control. In addition to its medical and emotional concerns, it is the wellspring of energies from which theories of personality and the growth of civilizations are derived. It is behavior which can be taboo, sacred, flaunted, sinful, illegal, perverted, and commercialized.

"If any man shall add unto these things, God shall add unto him the plagues that are written in this book" (Revelation of St. John the Divine).

But, sex can also be fun. It can be personally enriching. It can be a growth experience.

This book *closes* with its dedication: To Sexual Health.

Editor

Index

247